Mental Health and Inequality

Mental Health and Inequality

Anne Rogers and David Pilgrim

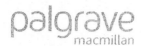

palgrave
macmillan

First published 2003 by
PALGRAVE MACMILLAN
Houndmills, Basingstoke, Hampshire RG21 6XS and
175 Fifth Avenue, New York, N. Y. 10010
Companies and representatives throughout the world

PALGRAVE MACMILLAN is the global academic imprint of the Palgrave Macmillan division of St. Martin's Press, LLC and of Palgrave Macmillan Ltd. Macmillan® is a registered trademark in the United States, United Kingdom and other countries. Palgrave is a registered trademark in the European Union and other countries.

ISBN-13: 9780333786567   hardback
ISBN-10: 0-333-78656-4   hardback
ISBN-13: 9780333786574   paperback
ISBN-10: 0-333-78657-2   paperback

A catalogue record for this book is available from the British Library.

A catalogue record for this book is available from the Library of Congress.

Library of Congress Catalogue Code Number: 2002042821

Printed and bound in Great Britain by
Antony Rowe Ltd, Chippenham and Eastbourne

Contents

List of figures, tables and boxes

Acknowledgements

The structure and content of the book benefited from the thoughts and input of Gill Bendelow, Mick Carpenter and Simon Williams (Department of Sociology, University of Warwick). We are grateful to Alistain Smith for feedback on Chapter 5 and to Jo Moncrieff for her comments on Chapter 8 about biological treatments in psychiatry. Anne Rogers in particular is indebted to Peter Huxley, Sherill Evans, Claire Gately, Richard Thomas and Brian Robson, who formed the research team of an ESRC-funded research project on Urban Regeneration and Mental Health undertaken jointly by the Institute of Psychiatry and the University of Manchester. The ideas that arose from joint discussions and from our research are particularly evident in Chapter 2. Research findings from two studies reported in Chapter 4 on primary care were shared with colleagues at the School of Primary Care and the National Primary Care Research and Development Centre at the University of Manchester (Carl May, Dianne Oliver, Linda Gask, Rod Sheaff, Martin Marshall, Steven Campbell, Susan Pickard, Shirley Halliwell, Martin Roland and Bonnie Sibbald). Finally, particular thanks go to Fran Morris for her efficient secretarial input. None of these people or organisations, however, should be held responsible for any opinions or mistakes that appear in what follows.

ANNE ROGERS
DAVID PILGRIM

Introduction

Recently, research on health inequalities has seen something of a revival, reversing a trend during the 1980s in which the existence of causal links between social conditions and health inequalities was questioned.[1] In the last five years, tackling health inequalities has assumed a prominent position both in research and in official health policy in Britain. However, mental health has received relatively less attention than physical health. Moreover, approaches to inequalities are spread across disciplines, which tends to fragment the object of our study. The theories and methods of medicine, psychology and sociology (to name just three contenders) are in tension, with partisan participants in a common investigatory field always at risk of mutual ignorance or of talking past each other.

A traditional public health approach to mental health not only rarely explicitly addresses the concept of inequality, its meaning is usually conflated, without question, with socio-economic disadvantage (cf. Macintyre 2000). Moreover, within this tradition, physical morbidity and mortality tend to be privileged and the problematic nature of medical knowledge applied to the study of emotional deviance is not explored. Public health medicine is a branch of medicine and so, unsurprisingly, its practitioners are professionally socialised into a commitment to the legitimacy of medical knowledge and reified DRGs (diagnostic-related groups).

Outside the public health tradition, within sociology, class and status have remained important but other politicised social variables, such as age, race and gender, have been increasingly considered. From this sociological tradition, the concept of inequality has also been problematised. Turner (1986) points out that to describe a differentiation of social roles (or 'social division') does not, in itself,

1

point to inequality. The latter only starts to take on meaning when evaluative analysis is introduced. In other words, versions of the notion of 'inequality' imply moral or political values, and coexisting ideological positions about inequality reflect and feed a tension between the societal values of individual freedom and social obligation in recent political debates and struggles.[2]

An emphasis on class and economic differences, with good reason, still predominates, but age, race and gender now regularly crosscut class, even if the latter remains centre-stage (Bartley *et al*. 1998; Graham 2001). A 'new generation' of health inequalities research has sought to extend traditional conceptualisations and research on health inequalities beyond that of the Black Report (DHSS 1980), which focused attention on three main theories of causation (artefact, selection, material).

Within this post-Black Report genre, there has been far greater attention paid to a fine-grained detail of the way in which aspects of social structure influence health risks (Blane *et al*. 1997). Also, it is clear now that social differentiation, rather than absolute levels of material and social resources, and the dynamics, as well as the character, of the social environment are important (Wilkinson 2000; Wilkinson, Kawachi and Kennedy 1998). The emergence of this new agenda has produced an interest in a complex relationship between a multitude of individual decisions, actions, and identities which reproduce social structure. There is a need to bring this new agenda into discussions of mental health and inequality.

What makes mental health special?

The peculiar weaknesses of psychiatric knowledge

The simple inclusion of mental health within health inequalities research is problematic on conceptual grounds. When examining the relationship between social position and mental health as dependent variables, conditions such as 'depression' or 'schizophrenia' are often assigned the same ontological status as, say, heart disease, diabetes or cancer as particular categories of morbidity. However, when mental illness is considered to be a medical condition, like any other, it brackets off the peculiar grime of mental health politics. In particular, it obscures psychiatry as a site of epistemological contestation and social control.

Whilst social constructivist critiques about physical health problems have blurred the distinction between physical and mental illness, such critiques have provoked a robust return to realism in the study of physical illness within medical sociology. Moreover, the physical diagnostic categories which have been 'picked off' more readily by radical constructivists are ones, like multiple sclerosis, with a contested aetiology (a shared vulnerability with the functional mental illnesses). As we will argue later, we prefer to address mental abnormality within a realist paradigm, but such an approach requires initially conceding the particular pre-empirical weaknesses of psychiatric knowledge. Whilst this does not imply an acceptance of psychiatric knowledge at face value (a naive positivistic stance), neither does it necessitate the wholesale rejection of the findings of psychiatric research as irrelevant pseudo-science.

Convincing arguments have been made that both physical and mental illness are ultimately defined by a sub-optimal social functioning. Also, many forms of common physical pathology, such as heart disease and cancer, are mediated by social and behavioural factors (for example, the health outcomes of population differences in dietary habits or tobacco and alcohol use). However, the issue is one of degree. The functional mental illnesses do not only (like, say, multiple sclerosis) suffer the problem of a lack of aetiological specificity and clear, uncontested, biological markers, they are also *particularly* sensitive to cultural variation, as psychiatrists studying their own nosologies discover (Kleinman 1988).

Whereas people with diabetes universally become weak and eventually die of ketone poisoning if they are untreated, this is not the case with those with a diagnosis of mental illness. The latter can be cared for paternalistically, wondered at, professionally labelled, ignored, sequestrated, valued or devalued depending on the social context. Under current social arrangements in Western society, of exclusion and impoverishment, madness certainly brings with it an increased risk of premature death, but it is not clear whether that correlation would be maintained if certain behaviours were valued and socially included. Certainly, there is evidence that rates of 'recovery' from 'schizophrenia' vary according to wider societal norms and responses to its amelioration (Warner 1985).

Disease categories, such as 'schizophrenia', have been subjected to persuasive conceptual and empirical critiques. The diagnosis has been criticised for its lack of aetiological specificity, its lack of predictive validity and its lack of inter-rater reliability (Bentall *et al.* 1988). Some historians of the concept (Boyle 1990) have even demonstrated that the symptom profiles recorded in the late nineteenth century, when Kraepelin and Bleuler invented the disease entity first called 'dementia praecox', and then 'schizophrenia', actually bear little relationship to the first-rank symptoms which psychiatrists currently use in the diagnosis. The features of patients and populations labelled as 'schizophrenic' were not the same as those with the same label today. Similar conceptual and empirical critiques can be levelled at the diagnoses of 'depression' and 'personality disorder' (Pilgrim 2001; Pilgrim and Bentall 1999). Thus, the methodological preoccupations of psychiatric epidemiology are chronically subverted by pre-empirical weaknesses in the profession.

Mental distress and conceptualising oppression

Another consideration about the peculiarity of mental health and inequalities relates to the conceptual issues debated by Turner (1986) about the meaning of 'inequality', i.e., not simply the categories of 'mental illness'. Social status and buying-power directly affect a person's sense of identity and thus directly constitute their sense of well-being. The term 'adversity' is commonly used in epidemiological studies about mental health. We use it episodically in this book but we recognise that it is problematic. The word can be interpreted as meaning 'misfortune of unknown origins'. This contrasts markedly with the term 'social injuries' preferred by writers such as Sennett and Cobb (1980). Their term embodies not only the outcome of exposure to noxious agents and the everyday grind of a poor life world, it also implies causes that are not randomly distributed in society. Instead, these reflect injustice and forces of oppression operating in a non-random way.[3] Thus, whilst oppressive conditions certainly negatively impact on physical health over time (hence the poor on average dying younger), a particular feature of mental distress is that it is the direct and immediate experiential consequence of these conditions. Objective forces of oppression generate concurrent subjective consequences of demoralisation and despair which are readily and misleadingly susceptible to medicalisation. There is another reason to attend to the peculiar status of mental health within the study of general health inequalities. Theorising about the latter has entailed great importance being attributed to social-psychological factors and the role of emotions as *mediators* in understanding physical health inequalities. Emotions have come to be seen as central to the relationship between social structure and health (Wilkinson 1996; Williams 1995). In relation to conditions seen as essentially physical, emotions are offered as a 'missing link' between physical illness and social structure. One consequence of this is that it leaves mental health as a condition more difficult to explore as an *outcome* of social conditions and particular personal contexts. What, if anything, mediates the relationship between social structure and mental health status, as an 'end' state, if the latter is now used generically as a *process* which explains inequalities in health? We would argue that mental ill-health should be considered as a set of outcomes, not merely relegated to a set of mediators of health status.

The social control of mental disorder

A further argument for separating out mental health from other conditions, for special consideration, relates to the different societal meanings and political responses that mental illness has evoked, compared to other forms of disability and deviance. In particular, the social origins of mental health problems need to be considered alongside the role of mental health services and the broader milieu which generates social disadvantage.

By the mid-nineteenth century, it became clear that madness was an important focus for the coercive State regulation of the poor. By the end of that century, asylums had transformed the character of the *lumpenproleteriat*, with a general decrease in officially recorded paupers being accompanied by an increase in people classified and detained in lunatic asylums. The category of madness spawned an extra layer of surveillance, containment and management which was not applied to those who were simply poor.

Historically, the mad have been a stigmatised group located in an ambiguous space between the deserving and undeserving poor. People belonging to this category were viewed as unable to contribute to economic productivity because of ill-health, and a label of emotional deviancy provided entry into the status of the deserving poor. However, unlike those with physical impairments or the old and frail, the mad were also feared and distrusted. Consequently, treatments viewed as 'scandalous' when imposed on the sane (detention without trial and physical intrusion on non-consenting bodies) have been deemed to be acceptable, both legally and ethically, for the 'insane'. The law, and psychiatric and public opinion have recurrently converged to sustain this double standard (albeit not without opposition).

The practicalities of regulating pauper lunatics, and their more recent equivalents, were entwined with particular theoretical assumptions about the medical nature of madness. Presumptions about the genetic origins of madness were rooted in theories about eugenics and biodeterminism. In turn, this theoretical position justified a somatic emphasis in psychiatric treatment, when the asylums rose and then declined. However, with the latter came strong theoretical and political challenges which still resonate today, first in 'anti-psychiatry' (Crossley 1998) and then in 'post-psychiatry' (Bracken and Thomas 1998).

The demise of the old mental hospitals during the mid-twentieth century and their gradual replacement with other forms of madness-management have not automatically brought about a reversal of the social divisions associated with the asylum system. Most psychiatric patients now reside outside large isolated institutions but a large number remain poor and socially marginalised. A key failure of modern mental health services has been their inability to break down the barriers of exclusion from economic and social life for those with serious mental health problems. For us, service provision represents an important and complex location for identifying and understanding influences of social and economic exclusion.

Equality of access to mental health services: problem or solution?

Health policy discussions about physical morbidity often focus on the need for greater access to care. There is a recurring sense in these debates that more (services) obviously equals better. However, mental illness is different as 'services' have been entwined with coercion far more often than has been the case with physical illness (Dallaire *et al.* 2000). Very occasionally, physical ill-health has been the basis for forcible sequestration. This can be contrasted with mental health work, which is involved with regular coercive control. Consequently, many people may not want to have more 'access' to mental health services but would rather have less contact or evade them altogether. Thus, the common political emphasis on equality of health service access does not apply neatly, if at all, to mental health services. The 'anti-psychiatric' emphasis, on valuing and respecting psychotic experience and letting madness be, was swimming against a tide of conservative public and professional preferences for greater 'imposed access' to psychiatric detention and treatment.

Recognising the extent of the social patterning of mental health problems in psychiatric knowledge

A final point we would make about mental health and inequalities relates to the psychiatric literature and its failure at times to acknowledge the social patterning of mental health problems. Although, within this literature, there has been a broad acceptance of the importance ascribed to 'the social' in ameliorating mental health problems, strategies for eliminating stigma and social exclusion may still obscure their social *genesis*. For example, a recent national campaign organised by the Royal College of Psychiatrists has aimed to reduce the stigma and discrimination experienced by people with mental health problems. However, this has entailed a spurious sense of *randomness* about mental health problems. This obscures their social patterning, divorcing mental illness from the social conditions which influence their incidence and prevalence. For example, the campaign announces:

> '1 in 4' reinforces the message that anyone can suffer from mental illness – '1 in 4' could be your brother, your sister. Could be your wife, your girlfriend ... 1 in 4 could be your daughter ... 1 in 4 could be me ... it could be **YOU**. (Website of the Royal College of Psychiatrists)

Our view, based on the evidence we summarise and appraise, is that these messages of randomness are misleading: one in four maybe, but not any one in four. This is not to imply that some psychiatrists are not fully aware of this fact. Social psychiatrists in particular have been central to its claim. However, the psychiatric profession is a broad church which is still dominated by biodeterminism and an expedient tolerance of the psychotherapeutic tradition in its ranks. As we will see in the last two chapters of the book, biological and psychological models converge to individualise psychopathology in the minds of most psychiatrists, and thereby obscure the social causes and consequences of mental health problems. As we will explore in our first chapter, expedient neutrality about aetiology within psychiatric knowledge has amplified and maintained social blinkers in the medical speciality.

The advantages of critical realism for exploring mental health and inequality

Bhaskar (1989) notes that it is the role of social science in its theoretical and practical work to explore and reveal the reality of the natural world, the events and discourses of the social world, and the structures which generate them. Critical realist thinking advocates a view in which it is not reality, which is socially negotiated, but our ways of conceptualising and investigating it. This theoretical and practical social science focus helps us to take a stance in this book. We do not limit ourselves (as the empirical realist or positivist may do, for example, in psychiatric epidemiology) to knowledge claims arising from specific observations. Instead, we can draw upon a range of findings and look for underlying processes which connect a variety of observations from different disciplines.

Fear and misery are ubiquitous and transhistorical physiological realities endured and experienced by humans and other animals. They are generated by an interaction of individual vulnerability and current or accumulated social and environmental insults and provocation. As for madness, as language-users embedded in particular cultures, human beings may break rules or fail in their role expectations in ways which are not intelligible to their fellows. Madness is defined by unintelligible conduct or speech judged in situated, cultural contexts. The mad break rules in ways that do not make sense to others *and* they produce no persuasive account for this unintelligibility to restore their credibility. They are convinced that they hear voices others do not or they hold fixed views about themselves, others and the world which are nonsensical to their fellows.

'Mental illness' may be a by-product of post-Enlightenment medicine, as emphasised by the Foucauldians, but *madness* is ancient and ubiquitous. We are not aware of any society, past or present, which has ignored or simply tolerated sustained unintelligible conduct. Even when it has been attributed with magical or religious power, rather than being dubbed a defect, its special nature has been acknowledged.

Given these assumptions on our part, we see little to commend reified concepts offered by most professionals, which overlay and seek a privileged status over basic lay descriptions of fear, misery and madness. At the same time, with all the imperfections of a reified and pretentious professional knowledge-base, psychiatric epidemiology still tells us much about the social derivation of recurring forms of deviance and distress. In this book we draw our conclusions from bodies of knowledge such as social psychiatry. The latter is predicated on categorical not situated reasoning (the patient 'has' schizophrenia, not the person is acting in an unintelligible way in this particular context). Nonetheless, if, say, 'schizophrenia' or 'depression' (medical labels) are taken as proxies for madness and sadness (social attributions), psychiatric knowledge still makes a contribution to sociological knowledge-claims.

However, for this utilisation of psychiatric evidence to work in the interests of social understanding, we need to invert a medical assumption for our own advantage. Whereas, psychiatrists believe that their diagnoses have a privileged epistemological status, vernacular descriptions or lay perspectives may be less mystifying (Coulter 1973; Rogers and Pilgrim 1997). For all its limitations, social psychiatric knowledge provides us with a database to discuss madness and misery in society. However, by taking a critical perspective upon this knowledge-base, we can both use its conclusions in a qualified way and situate psychiatric activity in its social context.

Critical realism (Bhaskar 1989) operates differently from naive realism, which presumes that mental illness and the diagnoses favoured by psychiatric professionals have a self-evident factual validity discovered by objective medical science, with cases to be counted and specific forms of patient pathology to be investigated. Psychiatric knowledge has developed in a social context that has been far from politically neutral. It has been legitimised by some interest groups and attacked by others, who have challenged the notion of a free-standing 'disinterested' or 'objective' body of medical knowledge which simply informs social research. Cultural and cross-national diversity pose a particular problem for psychiatric knowledge. On the one hand, modern psychiatry aspires to be universal in its authority about mental abnormality. At the same time, lay and professional judgements about the latter are situated in time and space.

A compromise has been made by 'comparative' or 'transcultural' psychiatry to claim the existence of two concurrent versions of psychopathology – the 'emic' and the 'etic'. The former alludes to culturally specific disorders and the latter to universal ones (Murphy 1982). Any substantial professional concession to the importance of 'emic' disorders threatens to undermine psychiatry as a universally applicable form of medical science, but to deny their existence immediately invites accusations of Western intellectual imperialism or racism. Rather than abandon their efforts at standard and universal forms of diagnosis as being ultimately futile, psychiatrists continue in their attempts to subordinate the emic to the etic (Cheng 2001), exposing them to these very charges.

The impact on mental health of place, culture and social divisions

Concepts that link agency and structure, such as 'cultural capital' and 'habitus' derived from the work of Bourdieu, have a particular relevance for our topic (Williams 1995). For this reason, we try to take into account a research tradition which highlights spatial differences (where people are) not just who people are, as well as their acquired knowledge and psychological competence and confidence, not just their economic circumstances.

In more recent times, the study of social divisions has been not only about social class, although, as we will argue for most of the book, this remains the most important of the defining dimensions of inequality. In some ways, differences in gender, or, strictly, biological sex, should be easier to investigate than class, which remains the subject of substantial conceptual argument within sociology as a whole, not just within medical sociology. Despite the apparently simpler territory of gender (the social face of sex), controversies remain about mental health differences between men and women, with feminist scholars being unable to agree even on whether women were, or were not, differentially oppressed by psychiatric services at their inception (e.g., Russell 1995; Showalter 1985).

Even when consistent findings have emerged about some forms of medically codified distress (such as higher rates of 'depression' in women), disputes occur about whether this is an artefact of measurement which is due to biological differences, or a function of socially created roles (Nazroo *et al.* 1998; Pilgrim and Rogers 1999). Similarly, any discussion of racial differences in mental health status can only proceed by examining a number of intersecting factors, including racism, the capacity of Western psychiatric knowledge to do justice to non-Western experience, immediate and distal impacts of migration and material differences between racial groups.

The structure of the book and the choice of material to analyse

In line with the assumptions outlined above, during the course of this book we will introduce considerations about material inequalities, social divisions, service responses and professional knowledge. The choice and ordering of the chapters we have included in the book reflect a number of ambiguities or tensions about our topic. As we have already noted, we give due respect to social psychiatric knowledge but also critically examine its limitations.

For now, we are riding on the back of a research tradition of psychiatric epidemiology, which at times naively promotes a trans-historical, universalising language of 'mental illness' or 'mental disorder'. In line with the critical realist perspective described above, where possible we try to situate the production of this in time and place. We acknowledge this most explicitly when looking at the relationship between violence and psychiatric knowledge (Chapter 6). Another pathway into this is the examination of one situated response to mental abnormality – the Western production during the twentieth century of 'mental health services'. The interrelationship between the latter and mental health is also construct specific. The focus of policy about violence and mental health has been targeted at those considered to have 'a severe and enduring mental illness'. The configuration of a primary care response to mental health (Chapter 4) has been predominately concerned with the so-called minor disorders of depression and anxiety. Being diagnosed with one rather than another diagnostic label certainly has differing implications for citizenship.

We will explore the duality of mental health services. The latter are *both* an aspect of a repressive State apparatus *and* a 'progressive' element of modern welfarism that, some of the time, provide an ameliorative response to distress and a secondary or tertiary preventive role. The latter may nip madness and distress in the bud or reduce the chances of their relapse, thereby reducing social disability. However, the clinical iatrogenesis associated with mental health services, which has been a spur for both professional dissent and disaffected user opposition, is palpable. Accordingly, we neither idealise mental health services, assuming that more equals better (the conservative professionalising position), nor demonise them (the abolitionist libertarianism of some user protest) but we do subject them to critical scrutiny.

A final ambiguity we work with is the assumption that it is not possible to capture a full picture of our topic unless we tack to and fro between an exploration of people with mental health problems in their social context and the current and historical activity, both practical and intellectual, of mental health professionals. This tacking will occur both within and between chapters. With these starting and organising principles in mind, the ordering of the chapters is as follows.

Chapter 1 describes and critically analyses contributions from two separate disciplines (sociology and psychiatric epidemiology) in mapping inequalities in mental health status. There are significant similarities between the two traditions. They share overlapping interests and have common historical origins. However, there are major differences between these currents of knowledge.

In **Chapter 2**, concepts of space and place are relevant to discussions of mental health and inequalities. We focus on the psycho-noxious influences in particular places on the genesis of mental health problems and the potential role of place in enabling and preventing recovery from mental health problems. The symbolic significance of placing people with mental health problems in particular localities is also explored.

Chapter 3 examines the credibility of the inverse care law for understanding variations in psychiatric service provision. We argue that a gradient of control in mental health services marks out mental health services from other mainstream health service provision. In this chapter, we begin to tease out the way in which mental health services and mental health status are related. We explore the ways in which theories about the cause of mental health problems are shaped and influenced by the configuration of service delivery.

In **Chapter 4**, we continue with a discussion of services and mental health but shift to an examination of primary mental health care. On the one hand, primary care has taken on a greater salience for people with mental health problems since deinstitutionalisation. On the other hand, primary care is discussed relatively infrequently compared to specialist mental health care. This contradiction has appeared at a time when technological changes and political expectations about primary care-led health services are ensuring a substantial period of clinical and organisational change. Drawing on two recently completed empirical studies,[4] we explore the way in which attempts to put the provision of high-quality mental health services on a par with other conditions have proved problematic.

In **Chapter 5**, we examine the evidence about social inequalities and the life-span. This evidence base reflects both the strengths and weaknesses of psychiatric epidemiology addressed in Chapter 1. Extensive cross-sectional and longitudinal studies have illuminated the nature of madness and misery during the life course, utilising medically codified knowledge (psychiatric diagnostic categories). Although this categorical approach is crude and has a tendency to be preoccupied with patient pathology (rather than professional activity), it still reveals important social patterns of relevance to the title of this book. Social psychiatry has made a legitimate contribution to our understanding of the social conditions which create, amplify or mitigate distress and dysfunction, and this chapter provides an overview of that contribution. By drawing upon recent work in realist medical sociology about the life course, we hope to summarise what we know about social disadvantage and mental health from infancy to old age.

In **Chapter 6**, the controversial relationship between mental health and violence is examined. Our starting emphasis is upon violence as a *source* of mental health problems (very much a minor theme in mental health policy). In the second part of the chapter, we then deal with the evidence about dangerousness and mental health status. It is clear in this chapter that not only has psychiatric knowledge been heavily shaped by a violent political context (warfare), but that political debates about patient violence still require a large injection of rationality. Whilst politicians may advocate evidence-based practice in mental health services (to improve efficiency), there remains much room for improvement in the production of evidence-based mental health policy.

In **Chapter 7**, we return to the question of professional activity. An aspect of inequality relates to the unequal power relationship which exists between professionals and mental health service users, about both knowledge and liberty. This chapter returns to a theme of the book about professional knowledge as a resource to understand inequality but also has an unequal power relationship. We also explore the nature of lay knowledge as a counter to traditional professional knowledge.

Chapters 8 and **9** continue this exploration by looking at inequalities in relation to biological and psychological treatments offered to or imposed upon people with mental health problems. The tension between conversational and somatic treatments is ancient but the most recent expressions of this tension reveal another set of important dimensions about inequality and mental health.

The above summary of our intentions in each chapter can be described in shorter form in Figure I.1, a triangular diagram of our three foci in the book.

The overarching aim of this book is to develop an extended framework of understanding of its title by examining the 'trialectic' relationships implied by the Figure I.1. We are aware that this requires us to criss-cross disciplinary boundaries. Readers of the book, within particular disciplines entered or drawn on, may feel that this journey does not pay enough respect to the legitimacy and depth of their conceptual assumptions or empirical resources. This is a price we have to pay for an attempt at inter-disciplinary inquiry.

We are aware that sociologists, in particular, have made elaborate contributions to the study of mental health. In its more populist expression, the discipline has even momentarily dominated public debates about the topic. The work of Goffman and Scheff comes to mind here and we draw on sociological ideas in a number of places. By contrast, social psychiatry has been, from its outset, an inter-disciplinary project, with psychiatrists conceding that psychologists and sociologists have often been in the methodological driving seat (Leff 2001). Unfortunately, what social psychiatry has gained in methodological rigour, it has often lost in its pre-empirical naivety.

This leaves us with two large chunks of knowledge. The first, from sociology, is highly theorised but not always easy, when on the outside of its disciplinary boundaries, to utilise. The second, from social psychiatry, is easier to understand, and more substantial in its cumulative empirical presence, but it lacks a critical reflexivity about the role of the mental health industry and the cogency of psychiatric knowledge.

Given the vast amount of knowledge already produced about social inequality and mental health from a variety of disciplines, we do want to digest and make sense of this for the interested reader new to the field. The task of originality we set for ourselves is to

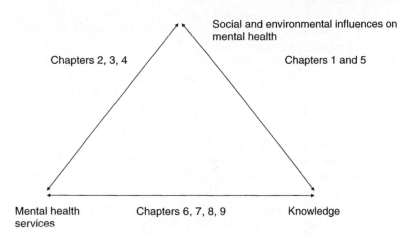

Figure I.1 The trialectic of services, knowledge and external influences

make a contribution to theory by exploring the trialectic relationship between social divisions, professional knowledge and the role of mental health services.

Summary

Here we summarise our assumptions and intentions in the book:

1 *No single discipline can make a persuasive claim of pre-eminence in the field.* We will draw upon the non-empirical and empirical work of several disciplines, including medicine, geography, psychology and sociology. We do not expect to deliver all of the academic expectations of any particular disciplinary perspective on the topic of mental health and inequality.
2 *Psychiatric epidemiology has made an important contribution in the field but critiques of psychiatric theory and practice undermine its legitimacy.* An interdisciplinary emphasis would not be required, or warranted, if psychiatric epidemiology had been persuasive to all of its readers. However, psychiatric knowledge has been hotly contested, both inside and outside of medicine.
3 *Mental health problems need to be explored as outcomes not just as mediators.* Whilst psychological factors have been explored as mediators of physical morbidity and mortality, this has led to

them being under-investigated as health outcomes. The book pays particular attention to this deficit.

4   *Mental health services play a part in the coercive and social control of deviance.* Mental health problems are different in many ways from physical health problems. Whilst the latter imply a norm of voluntarism during service contact, psychiatric inpatient facilities (and increasingly community interventions) are routinely involved in involuntary surveillance and control.

5   *The social control role of mental health services renders the notion of more equitable access problematic.* An implication of the previous point is that because mental health problems are met with a gradient of social control, it is not always clear whether increasing service access is a problem or a solution to individual patients.

6   *Mental health problems are socially patterned.* Mental health problems are not distributed in a non-random way in society. They reflect social divisons (of class, age, race and gender) and sometimes make a direct contribution to social inequalities (for example when patients suffer stigma and labour market disadvantage).

7   *Madness and distress are real.* It is not our view that it is sufficient to deconstruct professional representations of madness and misery. Mental health problems reflect real phenomena of fear, sadness and alienation from others. We do question though whether professional codifications of madness and misery are superior to lay views and understandings.

8   *An understanding is needed of the relationship between knowledge, services and causal antecedents of madness and misery.* Mental health and inequality can only be explored properly by avoiding forms of reductionism. In particular, the topic is not merely a matter of accepting professional accounts, or exploring equality of access to services (which are presumed to be benign and effective) or of only studying causal antecedents. It is the relationship between these three domains that is important, not any one in isolation.

1

Epidemiology and its limits

Introduction

In this chapter, we present some of the evidence about mental health inequalities generated by mainstream epidemiology. We do so principally to draw attention to the controversies which have surrounded the relationship between social conditions and mental health problems rather than to provide a comprehensive review of the evidence about inequalities and mental health.[1] We suggest, as others have done, that whilst traditional epidemiological approaches have illuminated relationships between social and psychological factors, explanations of causation are still weakly developed. This is because the development of knowledge in this area has been hampered by a number of tensions within psychiatric theory and practice and between psychiatry and social science. This tension has led over time to a gradual distancing of psychiatric epidemiology from other social scientific disciplines. This distancing has been a function of the development of distinctive disciplinary practices which have shaped restricted forms of scientific endeavour. We argue that this has undermined an adequate basis for mental health research. Our view is that psychiatric epidemiology has played an important part in producing evidence about the topic of this book but that its dominant role has left many unanswered questions and a poverty of theory about mental health inequalities.

Socio-economic status and social class

Epidemiology has furnished evidence about social class,[2] gender[3] and ethnic differences[4] in mental health status. The main methods of

17

psychiatric epidemiology have been the case series, the case-control study, the cross-sectional survey, the cohort study and the randomised controlled trial (RCT).

Despite changes in measures of both mental health and socioeconomic status (SES), the finding that higher prevalence rates for a range of mental health problems are to be found amongst those in the lowest social classes is firmly established. This cumulative evidence suggests that a strong inverse relationship with social class exists for those with diagnoses of 'schizophrenia', 'depression' (in women), 'antisocial personality disorder', 'alco holism', 'substance abuse', and 'non-specific distress'. Evidence about the relationship between lower social position and mental health is indicated by a recent systematic review of psychiatric epidemiology which echoes findings over the last 80 years. Fryers *et al.* (2001) found:

- A positive relationship between less privileged social position and mental health from five out of nine studies, with no studies showing an inverse relationship.
- A high income and material standard of living are associated with low rates of mental health problems, whilst low income and a poor material standard of living are associated with high rates.
- Poor education is associated with higher rates of common mental health problems in four out of six key studies.
- Unemployment, particularly recent unemployment (for both sexes), is associated with common psychiatric symptoms.

Most research on social inequalities and mental health has been conducted using measures of social stratification. Two broad conceptualisations have underpinned structural approaches to the study of social inequalities and mental health – social stratification and social class (Muntaner *et al.* 2000). Social *stratification* studies use measures of inequality which focus on disparities in social resources, such as years of education, occupation and income (Bartley *et al.* 1998). Social *class* research tends to refer to class locations originating from ownership and control over different types of asset (e.g., property and credentials). Aspects of the former approach include occupational, employment and housing status, income and wealth, and composite indicators. Occupational stratification is associated with differences in prestige, wealth, skills and working conditions (Blane 1995). Box 1.1 elaborates this point.

Occupational status

The use of occupational status in the UK was originally based on the 1911 Registrar General's Classification of Occupations which used the following definitions:

i.   Higher professional and managerial;
ii.   lower professional, technical and managerial;
iiinm.   skilled-non-manual workers and clerical workers;
iiim.   skilled manual workers;
iv.   semi-skilled workers and labourers;
v.   unskilled workers.

Classification of jobs by level of skill and social status is taken as an indicator of similarities across cultural, economic and environmental experience. Married women measured by men's occupation are also considered to share the same experiences. The use of classifications devised so long ago is problematic in establishing changes over time as structures and the status ascribed to particular jobs have altered considerably.

Box 1.1   Definitions and methods of measurement of socio-economic status

Employment status

Employed in economic activity and unemployment, which includes those seeking work, those not seeking work because of long-term sickness and/or disability, retirement. Divisions into period and duration of unemployment and those never employed.
   Changes in employment over time best measured by longitudinal design (cohort studies).

Education

Education is measured either as years of education (length of full-time education or age of completion of full-time education) or credentials (qualifications achieved). Its stability over adult life and reliability of measures are the reason for its popular use in psychiatric epidemiology. International comparisons are limited because qualifications and length of education are country-specific.

Housing

Housing status is considered to reflect wealth, income and social status. Housing status has been classified by: having a home or not (e.g., homelessness); type of house (flat, maisonette, terraced house, semi-detached, detached) and ownership status or tenure (social renting 'council' or owner-occupation). Area of residence and features of housing conditions (e.g., over-crowding) are also used in epidemiological studies.

Income and wealth

Broad income bands are used to measure individual and/or household income. The latter is considered the best indicator of material status for women. Material possessions are a common proxy for wealth and include home-ownership, access to a car and possession of domestic items.

Composite indicators

Indicators that reflect the multidimensional nature of social class, which encompass family income, personal educational achievement and occupational status.

Other factors associated with mental health symptoms and socio-economic status:

Disadvantaged life course status (e.g., being a single parent, having young children at home). Presence of absence of social support; life events; physical illness; activities of living include perceived loss of activity.

The relationship of disadvantaged social position to mental health differs according to the type of measure used. The strength of the relationship is weakest when using occupational grouping as the basis of comparison. A strong and consistent relationship between occupational status and mental health was evident up until the early 1980s (Dohrenwend 1990a). There has been less consistency in this finding since, which, in part, may be due to the decreasing relevance of traditional occupational status measures as an indicator of social position. Taken overall, studies indicate gender differences with a notably weaker connection evident between social class status and men's mental health (Fryers *et al.* 2000). There are stronger relationships between other indicators – education, unemployment status and income and mental health status. Box 1.2 summarises evidence about the relationship between class and mental health. However, the Fryers *et al.* review found that specific markers of social exclusion, such as being a single parent or having multiple illnesses, were better indicators of poor mental health than more general descriptions of social class or socio-economic status.

Box 1.2   Studies showing the strength of the relationship between occupational social class and common mental health problems in the UK (Fryers *et al*. 2000)

Health Survey of England 1998 (positive weak) A limited and inconsistent trend for mental health (measured using the GHQ12) to improve with increasing occupational social class (SCPR 1999)

National Psychiatric Morbidity Survey 1993 (positive) A clear social class gradient for neurosis amongst women (15% in SC I-II to 25% in SC IV-V) but far less for men, where all classes were similar except for SC I. (Weich *et al*. 1998)

Health and Lifestyle Survey (mixed, contradictory) No clear social class distribution: mixed results by gender and age (Hubbert and Whittington 1993)

British Household Panel Survey (positive) A clear negative gradient of measure of mental health with social class: those in lowest social class have highest prevalence. (Buck *et al*. 1994)

1946 Longitudinal Cohort Study (mixed, inconsistent) Higher rates of mental health problems in SC V compared to all others but not for men at age 36. (Fryers *et al*. 2000)

1958 Cohort (positive) Lower social class in both sexes show poorer mental health scores at age 23. Between ages 23–33 social class differences in scores diminish for men and increase in women (Manor *et al*. 1997)

Most studies summarised in Box 1.2 are of community surveys. Recently, a service-based sample was used instead (in primary care) (Ostler *et al.* 2001). From this study of 18,414 patients from 55 GP practices in Hampshire, England, the relationship between the siting of the practice and depression scores (age- and gender-adjusted) shows a clear relationship between depression and degrees of local deprivation. The importance of locality and services for mental health inequalities is returned to in Chapters 2, 3 and 4.

Causal models for mental health problems

Two main causal hypotheses have been put forward to explain the relationship between low SES or social class and poorer mental health: social causation theory and social selection theory.

Social causation theory

Environmentally oriented theorists (e.g., Bebbington *et al.* 1981; Brown and Harris 1978; Faris and Dunham 1939) suggest that higher rates of mental health problems amongst those of lower social class are due to a greater exposure to environmental and social stress. This includes living in poverty and deprivation, particularly in disintegrated communities characterised by social isolation, high crime and fragmented communication. In these communities, individual and community coping resources are both limited and chronically tested. A combination of external stressors with internal demoralisation and lack of personal control are offered to account for raised levels of madness and distress in conditions of poverty. Recent analysts have paid significant attention to relative deprivation and a gap between normative aspirations and the restricted avenues for realising these aspirations (Dohrenwend *et al.* 1998; Thomas *et al.* 2001).

Social selection theory

This suggests that social class is affected by mental disorder. Genetic and/or early environmental factors may be implicated in explaining the association between low socio-economic position and high rates of mental illness, either by increased vulnerability at times of stress or by simple biodeterminism (a biological 'time bomb'). It is important to note, then, that selection models do not focus *only* on genetic determination (see below).

A number of lines of inquiry have been pursued in order to explain the social class gradient in mental health, including experiences of family disadvantage in childhood, specific social-psychological and biological factors, and generalised vulnerability acquired though exposure to widespread adversity (Sacker *et al.* 1999). Explanations deriving from these broader categories have included class-based differences in foetal damage, genetic differences, stress, limited or inflexible conceptions of social reality and differences in coping mechanisms – all of which have been linked to 'lower social class' position.

Current debate

There has been an ongoing controversy about the social causation and social selection explanations. Although there has been some recent suggestion that processes of social selection and causation differ according to diagnostic type – for example, more persuasive evidence for social selection in relation to 'schizophrenia' and for social causation in relation to depression and anxiety (Dohrenwend *et al*. 1998) – in general terms there has been no definitive adjudication that one position is more compelling than the other. This is particularly the case in relation to the uncertainties about which variables (if any) are implicated in putative individual vulnerability.

Although sometimes the selection hypothesis has been mainly linked to genetic theories in psychiatry, logically social selection could occur as a result of early or aggregating psychosocial variables causing mental ill-health, which then culminates in individuals being socially disabled or incompetent. Hence, a neat dichotomy cannot be assumed, with the social selection hypothesis simply equalling a genetic position and the social causation hypothesis an environmental or social stress position.

This poses another problem in the debate, which is that vulnerability implies a relationship across time (from the embryo or childhood depending on whether a genetic or social learning position is favoured): a 'diachronic relationship'. By contrast, some social causation models emphasise moment-in-time adversity or trauma: a 'synchronic relationship'. Logically, of course, *both* diachronic and synchronic factors may have a causal relevance – hence the common consensus about 'stress-vulnerability'. Even within this inclusive logic, it still remains problematic to disaggregate the relative weighting or salience of different current and past variables.

The debate about social selection and social causation, being unresolved, has brought with it a set of uncertainties about mental health inequalities:

(1) Construct validity

The consistency of the social class gradient in relation to different psychiatric diagnoses appears to be less strong compared to physical illness (Sacker *et al*. 1999; Stansfield *et al*. 1998). Notwithstanding the increasing recognition of conditions which have inextricably linked components of psyche and soma, this may in part reflect *the lack of construct validity of mental illnesses* compared to physical illness. Even for those who do not dismiss mental illness as a myth and emphasise instead the functional criteria being present for illness (Szasz 1961; cf. Pilgrim and Bentall 1999), the construct validity and predictive validity of the major illnesses studied in psychiatric epidemiology, such as 'schizophrenia' and 'depression', are not robust.

(2) Longitudinal studies

With a few notable exceptions (e.g., Brown and Moran 1997; Johnson *et al.* 1999; Miech *et al.* 1999), a demonstration of the strength of the relationship between social position and mental health has been restricted by *the dearth of prospective longitudinal population-based studies*. These are necessary for an understanding of the development, interaction and impact of likely causal factors. For example, the likely presence of cumulative adversity through exposure to life events and stressful situations needs to be taken into account in making accurate assessments about mental health risk (Bartley *et al.* 1998).

(3) Psychiatric epidemiology

Despite a range of postulated causal explanations and some attempts, such as that by Brown and Harris (1978), which incorporate diachronic and synchronic factors, to provide sophisticated theoretical models, psychiatric epidemiology has remained underdeveloped theoretically, compared with other types of medical epidemiology and with predictive models in social science about social problems. There has been a tendency to engage in 'circular epidemiology', which is the replication of descriptive findings without attempts further to understand causation (Kuller 1999). Analyses which shed light upon the nature and meaning of the relationship between social class and mental health and illness have remained nascent or rudimentary compared to the study of physical health inequalities, and deviancy more generally, where causal theories have been more robust and there have been attempts to identify mediators of effect within a 'web of causation' (Kreiger 1994). For example, in criminology, which has also examined social selection and social causation processes as explanatory frameworks, there has been a substantial development of mixed selection-causation models. In support of social selection, low self-control in childhood was found to be predictive of disruptive social bonds and criminal offending later in life. In support of social causation, adolescent delinquency predicted later adult crime, and the impact of self-control on crime was mainly mediated by social bonds (Wright *et al.* 1999). In the mental health field there has been a tendency to attribute depression to social causation and for schizophrenia to be viewed as a result of social selection or 'drift'. However, analysis of SES as both a consequence and cause of mental health problems has only recently been seriously considered (Miech *et al.* 1999).

(4) Ideological difference

A major ideological difference between the social selection and social causation theorising is that the latter approach has been responsible for producing a more elaborate relationship between social influences and mental health than one concerned with social selection. This is associated with a greater optimism with a strong environmentalist assumption that changes in social conditions can influence mental health outcomes. Thus, the two positions are implicitly connected to political ideology – with the selection position being more conservative in intention, function or consequence.

Social processes implicated in mental health outcomes

The interconnection between low income, financial hardship, unemployment, poor housing and lack of education, which we can collectively call 'socio-economic adversity', could be corrected by political action. This recognition supports one of the ideological positions just noted. Traditional 'structural' approaches to mental health inequalities, such as the community studies of the impact of the environment on mental health conducted in the 1950s and 1960s (e.g., Hollingshead and Redlich 1958; Myers and Bean 1968), suggested links between socio-economic adversity and psychiatric morbidity. More recent research into the prevalence of mental disorder amongst women and the impact of poor employment, unemployment and a poor standard of living point to the importance of macro-structural variables and environmental causes in determining mental health (e.g., Warner 1985; Lewis *et al.* 1998).

In recent years, structural approaches to the study of mental health inequalities from the social causation perspective have been complemented by a literature on psychosocial factors, concerned with changes in, and the experience of, life events; the social world of individuals; and the way in which social environmental demands generate psychological stress (a precursor of distress and dysfunction) (Dohrenwend and Dohrenwend 1982; Elstad 1998).

The 'psychosocial perspective' refers to a number of related approaches which place a correspondingly greater emphasis on precipitating rather than predisposing factors. This offers potential policy cues for a reduction of the prevalence (rather than the incidence) of mental health problems. Take the example of poverty reduction as a mental health promotion policy. Although all social classes experience distressing negative life events, poorer people experience fewer positive life experiences to buffer them against these ubiquitous existential challenges. As the *ratio* of positive to negative life events is different in different social classes, a reduction in class differences would also reduce levels of psychological distress in a society (Phillips 1968).

Elstad (1998) distinguishes between approaches which examine the direct influences on psychological distress versus those where the influence is more indirect (e.g., when stress is expressed in health-damaging behaviour, such as violence or excessive consumption of alcohol and drugs). One of the most developed theories of negative stressors is the life events model, which encompasses the work of George Brown and his colleagues in relation to depression (Brown and Harris 1978). In mapping the social origin of depression, attention is drawn to three groups of interacting factors that produce depression (vulnerability factors, provoking agents and symptom formation factors[5]).

There has been some recent recognition of the need to view psychosocial influences as embedded in, rather than separate from, material influences (Stansfield *et al.* 1998). A link between personal agency and wider structural determinants of mental health is evident in a self-efficacy approach characterising the work of a number of social scientists interested in mental health (Aneshensel 1992; Mirowsky and Ross 1984; Pearlin 1989; Thoits 1995). An example is provided by an empirical study which explored people's responsiveness to specific environmental opportunities through highlighting the achievement, or blocking, of personal goals in maintaining mental health (Maas 1998).

Rather than viewing people as passive recipients of external circumstances (good or bad), the centrality of concepts, such as 'mastery', 'goal seeking', perceived control of the environment, and opposite notions, such as 'fatalism', and 'powerlessness', are important to examine in relation to changing 'opportunity structures'. The 'differential vulnerability' hypothesis proposes that not only are 'lower-class' individuals exposed to greater stressors, they are also more susceptible to their pathogenic effects because of a lack of resources such as social support and personal coping strategies. However, such theories have failed to adopt a context-specific approach in which aspects in the immediate environment might influence mental health outcomes. These are explored in greater detail in Chapter 3.

Gender and race differences

Whilst sex, like age, was frequently included as a variable in early epidemiological studies,[6] race and ethnic differences were not and, in the main, analyses of data focused firmly on social class differences. From the late 1960s attention turned to exploring gender and race and mental health as well as social class. Results on gender are tied closely to other key variables, such as social class, educational background and social circumstances.

As with more recent studies of social class, community studies have been used to explore gender and race and mental health. Community studies aim to provide information by measuring the level of mental disorder in society at large, independently of any contact people have had with services. The findings of these studies have been used to suggest that women experience relatively high rates of depression and other psychiatric disorders compared with men. Ground-breaking work was undertaken by Walter Gove and his colleagues (e.g., Gove 1972; Gove and Tudor 1972) focusing on the higher female rates among married women than men and a number of studies since that time have identified differences in female rates of mental health problems compared to men. As a result of this and subsequent work (e.g., Kessler *et al.* 1994; Pearlin 1975), one of the most consistent epidemiological findings is that of a greater prevalence of depressive disorders and 'non' specific psychological distress in women.

A 1958 cohort study suggested that between the ages of 23 and 33, social class differences in mental health scores diminished for men and increased in women (Manor *et al.* 1997). Additionally, the First UK National Household Psychiatric Survey has shown that women have a higher rate of neurotic disorder. This was highest in social classes IV and V and lowest in social class I (see Chapter 5).

A recent systematic review attributed gender differences in mental health scores to a range of social, familial and personal factors. These included: adverse experiences in childhood and adolescence creating anxiety and depression; socio-cultural roles and associated adverse experiences; psychological attributes which predispose individuals to negative life events and individual differences in coping skills (Piccinelli and Wilkinson 2000). Despite the findings of the review, explanatory factors focusing on social-psychological aspects are far from agreed. For example, a dedicated study set up to explore social role differences between men and women found that neither the number, or occupancy, of traditional 'female' caring or domestic roles accounted for gender differences in depression between men and women (Kessler *et al.* 1994; Weich *et al.* 1998).

Whilst there has been considerable interest in drawing out the differences between men and women, this tends to underestimate the similarities that remain between men and women in relation to mental health status. The latest Health Survey for England (1993–1998) showed that there was a tendency for mental health scores (using the General Health Questionnaire (GHQ)) to be correlated with social class in *both* men and women. Similarly, levels of functional psychosis reported in the First UK National Household Psychiatric Survey showed very high rates in social class V in both sexes. Some research shows the reverse in relation to gender. Analysis of findings in the 1946 cohort study PSE, last followed up in 1991, found that the highest PSE scores were in men not fully employed, from the lowest occupational social class, and renting their own home (Fryers *et al.* 2001).

In general terms, the specific discussion of male mental disorder is rare compared with the literature on women's mental health problems. An exception is the literature on male unemployment. The focus on female mental health problems also has the effect of underestimating the prevalence and content of male mental health problems and of the relationship between men and women more generally. The overrepresentation of women in depressed populations is well reported in the literature but the fact that *unmarried men* are also overrepresented and the possible origins of this finding are not widely discussed in epidemiological research.

The tendency in the literature for depression to be portrayed as an essentially female problem is also problematic. There are a number of studies which seem to provide evidence in absolute terms of higher rates for women. However, male depression is comparatively underexplored. There are reportedly high rates of suicide in young men, which is likely to be one outcome of psychological distress (the rates of suicide being higher in those with severe depression and psychosis) (Appleby *et al.* 1999). Higher suicide rates in young males may in part be due to their lack of ability or willingness to articulate distress (compared to young women). We examine suicide further in Chapter 6.

Gender differences in reporting may also account for a bias in the research of depression, with women being more ready than men to disclose the symptoms of depression to researchers. For example, in their ground-breaking work, Brown and Harris (1978) were quite explicit that their choice of a female-only sample stemmed from a gender assumption 'that women, who are more often at home during the day, would be more willing to agree to see us for several hours' (Brown and Harris, 1978: 49).

The gendered nature and relationship of mental health problems differ according to history, diagnostic category, cultural context and political origins and are reviewed elsewhere (Barnes and Maple 1992; Pilgrim and Rogers 1999; Russell 1995). The focus on female psychopathology within psychiatry has been viewed as a reflection and extension of oppressive patriarchy; the concern with redressing this imbalance has feminist origins. Feminist analyses focused on illuminating the way in which assumptions about gender-infiltrated constructs of mental disorder are commonly attributed to women and the role of patriarchy in sustaining an oppressive system of psychiatric control over women (Chesler 1972; Penfold and Walker 1984; Showalter 1987). These theorists in turn have influenced the tendency in recent years for the sociology of gendered health inequalities to focus on female rather than male disadvantage and the term 'gender' has tended to mean '*women*'.

The relationship of ethnic and racial status to mental disorder has, like the relationship with gender, been inconsistent and less established and studied. There are a number of studies in the UK and the Netherlands which suggest that racial differences in mental health have been found for diagnoses of schizophrenia, substance abuse and depression (Eaton and Harrison 2000). However, these have been subjected to vigorous methodological criticism and more recent comprehensive community studies of race and mental health seem to contradict the picture painted by earlier studies.

In Britain variations between ethnic groups, reported in studies carried out some time ago, reported lower rates of depression for people originally from the South Asian sub-continent than the white majority population (Cochrane and Bal 1989) and higher rates of psychosis for people of Afro-Caribbean origin. A more recent, and the largest, systematic population-based study undertaken of the prevalence of mental health problems among ethnic minority groups in the UK does not fully support earlier work. This larger study suggests that Caribbean men do not have higher rates of psychosis than the white majority (Nazroo 1998). These findings resonate with US evidence of the association of race with mental health inequalities in two of the biggest epidemiological studies, the Epidemiologic Catchment Area Programme Study (Robins and Reiger 1991) and the National Co-morbidity Study (Kessler *et al.* 1994). These found neither a strong nor consistent relationship between race and mental disorder. Similarly, recent evidence for race, class and 'common' psychological problems (anxiety and depression) is more contradictory than earlier studies suggest. As with gender, this is a hotly contested area which is bound up with the constructs and methods that are used as well as the latent assumptions of psychiatric knowledge.

In the UK literature, there is a bias towards studying psychosis amongst Afro-Caribbean people and a lack of focus on the study of anxiety and depression. Moreover, within psychiatric epidemiology specifically there has been a tendency to conflate variables such as race and socio-economic status (i.e., treating race as a proxy for SES) or towards artificially isolating race, class or gender by testing only their independent effects. Such an approach has the effect of underestimating the separate contribution of either racial discrimination or socio-economic privilege to inequalities or of exploring synergistic effects of race, gender and social class (Schwabe and Kodras 2000).

However, for our purposes the important point is that patterns between social variables, such as race, class or gender, are only that. Moreover, findings about these patterns change over fairly short periods of time. Additionally, whilst there has been considerable success in identifying patterns (albeit changeable ones), *explanations* for why such differences exist remain contested.

The role of knowledge in the mental health inequalities literature

The failure to develop a more context-specific explanatory framework discussed above resides, in part, in the changing knowledge base of social science and psychiatry. Studies tracing the relationship between social disadvantage and mental illness implicitly accept the legitimacy of psychiatric knowledge, treating diagnostic categories such as 'depression' or 'schizophrenia' as unproblematic and focusing on the social causes of mental illnesses. Yet the question of *what* is being identified has also pervaded the contested nature of knowledge about mental health. From one perspective, the difficulties have been seen in methodological terms as trying to attain better construct validity akin to the difficulties of, say, measuring other epidemiological variables, such as hypertension (Fryers *et al.* 2001). Others have reflected on the influence of external social and economic factors on the content of explanatory models. Dohrenwend (1998) for example comments that the

> belief in the paramount role of genetic inheritance began to change, especially in the United States, under the impact of two major events: the stock market crash of 1929 followed by the Great Depression, and the US entrance into World War II in 1941. The Great Depression made it clear that a person could become poor for reasons other than inherited disabilities and research conducted during World War II showed that situations of extreme environmental stress arising out of combat and imprisonment could produce serious psychopathology in previously normal persons, some of it long lasting. (Dohrenwend 1998: 224)

Dohrenwend suggests here that economic and war conditions shape the development of psychiatric knowledge. We return to the shaping influence of warfare on psychiatric knowledge in Chapter 6.

Peacetime conditions between the two 'World Wars' of the twentieth century largely witnessed 'business as usual' with a biomedical approach in psychiatry returning to the fore. The shift from a biological to an environmental emphasis in the period Dohrenwend addresses went into reverse eventually. In the same year that Dohrenwend was making his historical point, we find the following confident statement from biological psychiatrists about their postwar triumphs in relation to 'the pathophysiology of schizophrenia':

> The discovery of anti-psychotic drugs, such as chlorpromazine and haloperidol, in the early 1950s, had a tremendous impact on the treatment of schizophrenia. Long-term inpatient stays became increasingly uncommon, and the challenges of treating patients with schizophrenia began moving from the inpatient to the outpatient arena.... However, the discovery of anti-psychotic drugs also had a major impact on our conceptualisation of schizophrenia. For the first time firm evidence [*sic*] existed that schizophrenia had a physical basis and that physiological models of intervention could be employed to treat the disorder. (Csernansky and Grace 1998: 185)

Here, we find a set of interlocking assertions and assumptions about biological causation and biomedical authority.[7] Such assertions have been disseminated more broadly in the public domain by commentators such as Edward Shorter (1997), who pronounced at the beginning of his book, entitled *A History of Psychiatry*:

> if there is one central intellectual reality at the end of the twentieth century, it is that the biological approach to psychiatry – treating mental illness as a genetically influenced disorder of brain chemistry – has been a smashing success. (Shorter *ibid.*: vii)

And yet, by the 1990s, *contra* Shorter, most psychiatric historians had come to a consensus that the 'pharmacological revolution' was, if not a myth, a considerable uncertainty (Scull 1979; Warner 1985).[8] The examples cited above from Dohrenwend, Csernansky and Grace, and Shorter highlight why psychiatric epidemiology has not merely been a technical, or methodological matter, it has also been an important site of ideological struggle.

Turning to assumptions and constructs within social psychiatric research, the questioning of objectivity and neutrality of central concepts of race, class and gender have in themselves become the focus of substantial critique. The latter has consistently pointed to the way in which these categories are 'socially constructed' or framed, which may result in the exacerbation, as well as the measurement, of inequalities in mental health. This is most evident in the study of differences in race and mental health where reification and the amplification of racist assumptions about different ethnic groups have permeated the inequalities in mental health literature. The way in which 'race' and 'culture' are inextricably bound up in the construction of disease categories is illustrated by a number of past and contemporary examples. For example, 'drapetomania' was defined by an American psychiatrist, Cartwright, in 1851 as a disease which made slaves run away:

> The cause in the most of cases, that induces the Negro to run away from service, is as much a disease of the mind as any other species of mental alienation, and much more curable, as a general rule. (cited in Ranger 1989: 354)

More recent examples are constructs of 'cannabis psychosis' and, for some, even the ubiquitous 'schizophrenia'. Until recently, 'cannabis psychosis' was a label attached selectively to Afro-Caribbean people when psychiatrists were perplexed by their behaviour (Ranger 1989). Psychosis was defined by the Royal College of Psychiatrists as a mental illness which 'cannot be understood as an exaggeration of ordinary experience'. Fernando (1988) points out the rise in racist categories is bound up with the institution of slavery and social control. Pilgrim and Rogers (1999) have suggested that the interest in dualistic reasoning between 'black and white' characterising race and mental health acts to accentuate and polarise differences. This is further accentuated when consideration is given to how the variables of depression and psychosis and their measurement are currently constituted.

In contrast to a traditional medical emphasis on diagnostic categories, a number of prominent social psychiatric researchers have advocated a dimensional view, in which there are gradations of psychological distress (Goldberg and Huxley 1992). This has filtered down into common tools such as the General Health Questionnaire (GHQ) commonly used in primary care and community population surveys.[9] The relevance of this for race is the reinforcement of a dichotomy between a negative highly stigmatised and medicalised category, such as 'schizophrenia', and its association with ethnic identity at the same time as a rapidly demedicalised and normalised view of anxiety and depression and its measurement has emerged which is relatively less frequently associated with race.

Three generations of research into mental health inequalities

Conducting and appraising isolated epidemiological studies can distract us from the way in which disciplinary knowledge takes shape, consolidates and changes over time. 'Methodologism' inherent to the recent norms of much epidemiology can generate a version of 'superficial empiricism' which is neither theorised nor reflected on. Avoiding this distraction or tunnel vision, and standing back from the field, Dohrenwend (1998) identifies three distinct generations of mental health inequalities research that have been accompanied by 'dramatic changes in psychiatric nomenclature' (Dohrenwend *ibid*.).

First-generation studies covered the period up until just after the Second World War in which hospital samples and clinical diagnoses were used to describe the patterning of mental illness. Mental health and public health reform movements originating in the nineteenth century were imbued with a moral and reforming thrust aimed at the poor. The division between the way in which the social and environmental causes of physical health were dealt with contrasts with the attention given to mental health. In the former, the connection between poor living conditions and ill-health was a salient feature of the origins of epidemiology and public health as a medical discipline.

The identification of the relevance of structural, environmental and social conditions is vividly conveyed by the accounts of Rudolph Virchow in 1848 identifying the poor living conditions of the people of Upper Silesia as the cause of illness (Tesh 1990). Another illuminative event was of TV reporter John Snow removing the handle from the parish pump to eliminate an epidemic of cholera. Important public health measures mirrored this concern with the introduction of population-based interventions, which were overlaid by the pursuance of policies characterised by social justice. Water and sewerage were regulated, factory and housing conditions improved through legislative action, and child labour was abolished.

The focus of Victorian psychiatric epidemiology was, in a major respect, different from mainstream medical epidemiology, being concerned not with removing a pathogenic source of community contagion but with institutional populations and segregation. Psychiatric epidemiology began (and in many ways continues) with a preoccupation with counting cases of mental disease, not with mapping sources of pathology (as these are predominantly unknown). Whereas infectious agents were the concern of medical epidemiologists, psychiatrists were more concerned with the assumed genetic threat of pauper lunatics. In the late nineteenth century, Lunacy Commissioners used the epidemiological approach in mapping and commenting on the distribution of insanity across populations in their efforts to construct a separate psychiatry for the poor. The massive expansion of the lunatic population was fed almost totally by the pauper insane. Over the same period, private patients hardly increased in numbers at all. Psychiatric epidemiology was bound up with a broad eugenic social policy of segregating an assumed 'tainted' gene pool (see Porter 1989; Scull 1979).

The demographic analysis of an institutionalised mentally ill population reached its peak in the USA during the 1920s. It was not until the late 1930s and 1940s that greater importance was assigned to social inequalities in psychiatric and social epidemiology. In these early studies, investigations depended, in large part, on key informants and agency records. Studies based on direct interviewing produced low prevalence estimates. Armed with advances in epidemiology, including the use of new statistical and sampling techniques, subsequent studies turned their attention to surveying broader groups in the population and examining the role of environmental variables and the incidence and prevalence of mental illness in the community (Dohrenwend 1998).

The second phase of epidemiological studies involved the development of human ecology as a theoretical trend within the Chicago School of sociology (Pilgrim and Rogers 1994). At the outbreak of the Second World War, a prominent study based on social ecology and entitled *Mental Disorders in Urban Areas* was published by members of the Chicago School (Faris and Dunham 1939). Keen to show the influence of poverty and deprivation, they contrasted the prevalence of manic-depressive psychosis, which appeared to be randomly distributed across the city of Chicago, with the numbers of people diagnosed with schizophrenia found predominantly in poorer areas. Whereas Faris and Dunham focused on social isolation as a possible aetiological factor, Hollingshead and Redlich reflected the popular appeal of Freudian ideas, which were prevalent in the USA at that time, in their subsequent study. They suggested the influence of social factors that spanned the life course and emphasised the experience of early infancy.

This second generation of research on inequalities in mental health began to follow those evident in mainstream public health with a focus on environmental conditions and the quality of interpersonal relationships in different parts of society. Subsequently, a range of influential studies identified the relationship between mental health and social class and demonstrated a consistent social patterning of mental disorders. These studies showed that rates of mental health problems were more prevalent amongst those in the 'lower' classes (e.g., Hollingshead and Redlich 1958; Srole and Langer 1962). Consistently reported findings were that the diagnoses of schizophrenia and personality disorders were inversely related to social class. For so-called 'common mental health problems ('anxiety and depression') a link between social disadvantage and mental health was also established, although this appeared to be less consistent than the finding for schizophrenia (see below). The trend for affective psychoses (e.g., 'manic depression' now called 'bi-polar disorder') was towards greater prevalence in 'middle-' and 'upper-class' populations.

Over the past thirty years, the third generation of studies has returned to its original focus – the mental institution and the mapping of population need to match service provision. The emergence of a policy of community care (very slowly from the 1930s) brought with it the need to enlarge surveillance associated with the increased medical management and risk reduction in those considered most vulnerable. This, most recent, phase has been characterised by greater diagnostic specificity and case identification which accord with the 'medical necessity' for intervention. This can be contrasted with the preceding phase which had been more concerned with the identification of the root causes of mental health problems in social environments. Currently, policy and practice imperatives remain firmly rooted in a concern with identifying rates of diagnosed mental illness in populations in order to provide sufficient specialist services. This has largely displaced the community environment focus of studies in the second generation, although in some studies *both* strands of interest can be found.

The relationship between sociology and psychiatric epidemiology

The broad professional aspiration of social psychiatrists has been to join a wider project of medical epidemiology. According to Williams *et al.* (1986) the attraction of epidemiology is that it seeks to address the problem of disease in the context of the community as a whole. Traditionally, the aims of psychiatric epidemiology have been identified as being concerned with definition, aetiology, natural history, treatment and outcome of disease. In particular, the following functions are emphasised:

- The completion of the spectrum of diseases
- The establishment of outcome
- The actuarial assessment of morbidity risks
- The evaluation of the efficacy of treatment
- The conceptual construction of diagnosis/classification.

During the second generation of research noted above, a strong alliance with sociology was evident in pursuing the above agenda, and social scientists were active members of academic departments of psychiatry (Klerman 1989). This close association between epidemiology and sociology is traceable to nineteenth-century social medicine (Kleinman 1986; Rosen 1979) which grew in the twentieth century, with sociologists joining psychiatric epidemiologists in seeking to identify the causes of mental health problems and linking these back to social and material conditions. The growth in legitimacy of psychoanalysis in the 1930s and 1940s, and the consequent acceptance of 'continuum' models to add to, rather than wholly displace, the traditional categorical approach in medicine, made the lack of precise classification acceptable to both psychiatry and sociology. Moreover, in relation to secondary and tertiary prevention, fruitful alliances were made with social scientists that tied the subject of mental health firmly to the social. For example, this included research into the role of adverse and alienating conditions within mental hospitals in exacerbating or amplifying *existing* mental health problems – 'institutionalism' (Brown and Wing 1962). This phenomenon had been identified earlier as 'institutional neurosis' (Barton 1958) and now tends to be called 'institutionalisation'.

Such studies ensured that sociological knowledge, with its direct connection to inequality and the social nature of mental health problems, permeated the discipline of psychiatry. A mutual and fruitful relationship characterised the relationship between sociology and psychiatric epidemiology, as indicated here by Lawson (1989), a sociological contributor to social psychiatry:

> Psychiatry accepted that, as its disease categories were so tenuous and not generally marked by physical signs, the sociologist's concepts of impairment or disability marked by social dysfunctions could be the key to unravelling the rates of mental illness. (Lawson 1989: 38)

Whilst sociological work grounded in epidemiology has continued, there has also been a retreat from the relationship with social psychiatry. After the late 1960s, there was a redirection of sociology away from positivism and a broad openness to other orientations. This was important in two respects. The tradition of symbolic interactionism (from another part of the Chicago School) and newer trends such as ethnomethodology and social constructivism brought distance into the common ideological project of social engineering, which had previously acted to cement the enterprises of medical sociology and social psychiatry.

A set of different studies with a radical departure emerged. This included work inspired by the distinction Lemert (1967) had made between primary and secondary deviance and its elaboration in the 'social reaction' theory of Thomas Scheff (to be better known imminently as 'labelling theory'). From this point on, psychiatric illness was treated with suspicion by sociologists and their interest turned to the social processes which led to labelling and diagnosis and the social consequences of psychiatric practice.

A further sociological project emerging after the late 1970s was represented in the study of changes in the discursive practices of psychiatry attributed to a postmodern society, a branch of work considerably influenced by French poststructuralism (Foucault 1965; Prior 1991; Rose 1990). Whereas the previous relationship between psychiatry and sociology had been built on cooperation or common understanding, or at least an ability to ignore or tolerate epistemological differences, these newer studies were explicitly critical not only of psychiatry but also of the constructs which constituted the subject matter of psychiatry and epidemiology (Pilgrim and Rogers 1994). Such a shift was understandably met with counter-arguments and resentment from psychiatrists who had previously gained much from their collaboration with sociology and from the analysis of social forces (e.g., Wing 1978).

Another effect of this change from within sociology was pragmatic rather than ideological. Psychiatrists had previously accepted that social scientists had particular methodological expertise (Lawson 1989). In its Durkheimien form, sociology presented itself as an objective project whose purpose was to study social problems and produce knowledge which could be used to further policy objectives. However, later sociologists wished to show how mental illness was socially negotiated, constituted or constructed, as well as exploring its connectedness with everyday norms and values of society and the deployment of psychiatry as a means of social control. By contrast, social psychiatry became increasingly concerned with establishing invigorated and technically robust constructs of mental illness and elaborating methodological rigour. Sociology was in many ways undermining the professional credibility of psychiatrists, at the very time when they were becoming more entrenched in a medical–scientific paradigm.

This diverging agenda brought a substantial distance into the relationship between sociology and social psychiatry. Wing, an eminent social psychiatrist who had worked closely with sociologists (e.g., George Brown), chided psychiatry for a failure of scientific practice in the face of the onslaught of criticism that came from labelling theorists such as Scheff. Writing in 1979, Wing argued for the establishment of a narrower set of scientific categories of disease, which he saw as essential for psychiatry to distance itself from lay constructs of madness and popular contemporary critiques of the legitimacy of the concept of mental illness and the role of psychiatry in society. Wing suggested:

> One reason why medical practices have come under criticism in recent years is that some psychiatrists use a term like schizophrenia in a non-technical, virtually a lay sense and make and act on a diagnosis when there is not reason to suppose that a disease theory can usefully be applied. The broader their concept of 'schizophrenia' the more liable they are to make such mistakes. (Wing 1978: 164)

This concern expressed by Wing pointed up a long-standing epistemological problem for epidemiological studies in psychiatry, which was the imprecision of classificatory systems (nosologies) compared to other medical specialities. Earlier, Elfkind (1938) had commented in a leading American epidemiology journal that data based on psychiatric diagnostic categories implicated 'more or less intangible concepts, because psychiatry, dealing so much with the mind, must perforce concern itself with subjective experience, which is so difficult for scientific study and analysis'. Later, Eaton emphasised this inherent contradiction, namely:

> Epidemiology is a branch of medicine and thus the assumptions of the medical model of disease are implicit. The most important assumption is that the disease under study actually exists. In psychiatry this assumption is assuredly more tenuous than in other areas of medicine, because psychiatric diseases tend to be defined by a failure to locate a physical cause, and a validation of a given category of disease is therefore more subtle and complex. (Eaton 1986)

Screening measures used in second-generation population surveys recorded aspects of non-specific distress or, as Dohrenwend termed it, 'demoralisation'. This included a response to chronic physical illness, recent life events, or being in a low-status social position. Dohrenwend and colleagues estimated that non-specific distress occurred with a frequency approximately equal to that of 'diagnosable psychiatric disorder'. If social psychiatry aligned itself with social scientists and retained an allegiance to the notion of mental distress as a continuum of vulnerability (typical of second-generation studies), this was not a problem. However, it did become an issue when social psychiatry and epidemiology became estranged from sociology during the third generation of research.

In recent years, psychiatric epidemiology has been preoccupied with description and measurement of mental disorder, which has been viewed as a precursor to the future project of advancing analytical and experimental epidemiology. The development of reliable and valid structured diagnostic interviews, deployed in cross-national surveys of the prevalence and correlates of mental disorders, have featured strongly in this agenda.

From the 1980s onwards, there was a concern with developing more robust measurements and categorisation of mental health problems. In particular, there was a greater use of survey interview methods designed to diagnose a variety of 'mental illnesses' leading to accurate population estimates of the prevalence and incidence of specific disorders (Kessler *et al.* 1994). More recently, epidemiological research has been seen as a means for strengthening the links psychiatry has with the neurosciences, clinical research and public health. In other words, the emphasis has been on medicalising the project of psychiatric epidemiology.

Extending the range of design and methods beyond the emphasis on large-scale cross-sectional and general population studies, according to some, will allow a broader spectrum of psychopathology to be studied. The latter is intended to include an inquiry into 'etio-pathogenic' processes (genetic, neuroscientific and psychological factors) for the onset and persistence of psychopathology (Wittchen 2000). This speculative biopsychological emphasis stands in opposition to both the previous focus on the social conditions of individuals and the concern with levels of demoralisation amongst community populations.

A preoccupation with standardising and refining descriptive diagnostic categories also replaced the tendency of previous generations of research to pioneer their own methods and procedures for case identification. Whilst this might have meant that little attention was given to problems of validity, it had allowed the proliferation of psychoanalytic and other biographically inspired models. These allowed personal experience and inner life to become windows into the social world. The categories of DSM-1 and 2 were heavily influenced by both psychoanalytic theory and wartime social psychiatry (Carpenter 2000).

Later shifts in DSM and the section on mental disorders in the International Classification of Diseases (10th revision) brought about major changes in case identification and classification. DSM II, whilst not adhering to what may be viewed as explicit social aetiology, nevertheless incorporated psychoanalytically influenced ideas about aetiology. By contrast the specific aim of moving to DSM III was to expunge causality from diagnosis in favour of behavioural *description*:

> Because DSM III is generally atheoretical with regard to aetiology, it attempts to describe comprehensively what the manifestations of the mental disorder are, and only rarely attempts to account for how the disturbances came about, unless the mechanism is included in the definition of the disorder. This approach can be said to be descriptive in that the definitions of the disorder generally consist of descriptions of the clinical features of the disorders. These patterns are described at the lowest order of inference necessary to describe the characteristic features of the disorder. (DSM III 1980: 7)

Subsequent changes from DSM III to IV represent a further progressive elimination of patient subjectivity and their biographical and social context, in favour of an antiholistic model of mental illness compatible with biological psychiatry (Mishara 1994; Wallace 1994). Above, we noted Dohrenwend's observation about the history of psychiatric epidemiology, that models of mental health inequality research represent an interaction of the internal focus and the dynamics of the discipline of psychiatry with the *zeitgeist* of the wider social economic and political milieu. Echoing this, Carpenter (2000) views this trend of promoting standardised categories of normality and disorder in DSM as part of a US-inspired 'Mac-Donaldisation' of social and economic life.

From this perspective, DSM IV represents 'the psychiatric equivalent of the World Trade Organization (WTO), promoting the principles of American Universalism as objective standards that are beyond reproach' (Carpenter 2000: 615). Certainly one of the consequences of this focus on narrowing measurement and objective criteria has been a negation of the consideration of context and experience as part of the epidemiological endeavour. Whilst qualitative sociology in studies of disadvantage in other areas have shed light on issues of cultural identity and discovered highly complex sets of social relationships, in epidemiological work about mental health this has been a missing element and in the UK is only just starting to be reconsidered.

A crisis in the study of mental health inequalities

Despite the multiple sources of evidence about the social origins and consequences of mental health problems, by the end of the twentieth century inequalities in mental health research were weakly represented in a research context where greater emphasis was being given to social inequalities in health as a whole (Muntaner *et al.* 2000). At present, not only is there less research (compared to the study of physical illness) but causal explanations and frameworks about the inverse relationship between mental health and social position remain underdeveloped. We have argued above that this current poverty of theorising has been driven, in part, by a historical legacy which took sociology and psychiatry down different paths. The mutual project of social psychiatry and sociology which mapped the social causes of mental pathology collapsed when sociological concerns turned towards showing the way in which traditional psychiatry and mental health services contributed to the marginalisation of those labelled as being 'mentally ill'. These criticisms also focused on the way in which constructs of mental illness central to the enterprise of psychiatry were imbued with stigmatising, coercive and ideological intent.

Whilst social psychiatry turned its attention to issues of ensuring greater validity and reliability for the diagnostic constructs, which were construed as central to its lack of scientific credibility, sociology turned its attention to the social and political nature of psychiatric practices. One partner became introverted and the other more hostile, creating a vicious circle. Only those sociologists (and psychologists) who were prepared to accept psychiatric knowledge uncritically remained within the inter-disciplinary alliance, which had become 'social psychiatry'.

Whilst more robust methods and credible diagnostic constructs arguably have been the product of recent psychiatric epidemiology, they have been at the expense of a more sophisticated understanding of the social nature of mental health inequalities. For example, a recent study found that the subjective rating of quality of life for individuals in a residential population was associated with levels of distress which would not normally be counted as constituting either a major or minor mental illness (Thomas *et al.* 2002). This important reminder of low-grade unhappiness and demoralisation as part of a continuum of distress and dysfunction can be contrasted with an emerging rigid categorical world of the third generation of psychiatric epidemiological studies. In this third generation of research, social psychiatry may have raised its credibility in the eyes of medical colleagues in other specialities but it has taken it away from social science and the rich potential offered by the latter.

The bias towards a medicalised view of the relationship between mental illness and social position has also demoted or obscured a view of what the levels of psychological distress in a society suggest about its character. The level of distress amongst community populations is a marker of social progress, levels of current alienation and the success, or otherwise, of social policies designed to improve the quality of life of its citizens. Levels of psychological distress are also markers of the extent of relative deprivation in a society and its political health. The third generation of an overly medicalised form of epidemiology obscures rather than illuminates our social and political life world.

Take the example of recent changes in Eastern European societies. Massive rises in suicide, alcohol consumption and violence have been brought about by social and economic upheaval in their social orders. There is a consensus in public health quarters that these are essentially social in nature (Tkatchenko *et al.* 2000) and that inequalities in physical illness are mediated by psychosocial factors (Wilkinson 1996; Williams 1995). Mental health states, in themselves, are also worthy of separate consideration as the outcome of social processes, influences and context and, conversely, as reflections of social advantage and disadvantage in a society. In the next chapter we examine the increasing importance of understanding neighbourhood when understanding social divisions and inequalities in mental health.

2

Neighbourhood, community and mental health

Introduction

During the 1930s, there was an enthusiastic focus by researchers, particularly those in the USA, on neighbourhood, which shaped early epidemiological studies. The problems created by the economic depression gave rise to a number of studies of geographically specific communities. Subsequently, a strand of social psychiatric epidemiology continued to include reference to context and place in exploring the impact of extreme situations on mental health. This work examined, for example, the impact and legacy of the Holocaust (Levav and Abramson 1984), the Cambodian tragedy (Mollica *et al.* 1993) and a range of natural and human-made disasters (Geil 1998).

Notwithstanding these contributions, the influence of ordinary neighbourhoods on mental health has not been comprehensively tracked over time and place. This source of influence has remained in the conceptual shadow of key socio-economic, individualised and symptom variables discussed in the previous chapter. However, more recently there has been a growing recognition that policies designed to make improvements to the physical and social infrastructure of localities might contribute to the reduction of socio-economic gradients and that what constitutes an individual's socio-economic status is, to an extent, entwined with the conditions of life in their locality (Graham 2001). Macintyre *et al.* (2001) have argued that a greater understanding of how people actually live in their homes is required to arrive at a perspective of 'residency as a relational resource and experience'. In relation to mental health specifically, there are arguments for understanding resilience to psychological stress through exploring what goes on within communities

45

and the way in which individuals adapt to and interact with their environment.

Recently, there has also been a return to the focus of the early Chicago School studies, with 'locality' assuming a greater profile in analysing the fate of those discharged from the old mental hospitals and the quality of life of those living with long-term mental health problems 'in the community'. The disappearance of asylum walls has resulted in a reunification of pauper lunatics with other lowly regarded social groups. Research has illuminated an uneven dispersal of those with mental health problems across social space. In a number of countries, there has been a concentration of those with mental health problems in areas with high rates of poverty, social disorganisation, substance abuse and criminality.

In the light of these introductory comments, this chapter has three aims:

- First, we explore the way in which the genesis of mental health problems, particularly in urban environments, has been conceptualised. Whilst we recognise the specific effects that rurality might have on mental health need, we focus on urban environments because of their seemingly greater relevance to inequalities. The considerable British urban–rural differences in mental health (which show higher rates of psychiatric morbidity, alcohol and drug dependency in urban areas) have been assumed to be largely attributable to more adverse urban social environments (Paykel *et al*. 2000).
- Second, we focus on the treatment and management of those with mental health problems in community settings.
- Third, we explore the management of mental health problems in the context of locality and social policy.

The spatial distribution of mental disorder

Faris and Dunham's early epidemiological research inspired a proliferation of interest in the relationship between social position and mental illness and its connection with specific localities. Whilst no distinctive pattern across localities was found in relation to the spread of affective conditions, Faris and Dunham found high rates of schizophrenia and substance abuse 'in the deteriorated regions in and surrounding the centre of the city, no matter what race or nationality inhabited that region' (1939: 35). On the basis of this finding, they argued that the lack of social integration in socially disorganised communities contributed to the 'confused, frustrated, and chaotic' behaviours that typified the expression of many mental health problems.

Subsequent reviews of ecology and mental health confirmed consistent variations between urban areas differentiated by population size, social class and economic prosperity and between rural and urban areas (Giggs 1987; Smith 1984). Whilst the geographical plotting of 'treated' cases has been viewed as having considerable utility for planning mental health service provision, the contribution of the older Chicago-type studies for understanding and evaluating the impact of the urban environment on mental health status has been less evident. In many epidemiological studies conducted, there has been a continuing tendency to treat the socio-economic status of individuals as a proxy for the social contexts in which people live. This assumption has been challenged by evidence that neighbourhood seems to have an independent effect on mental health. For example, residents of disadvantaged neighbourhoods have shown a greater propensity to report symptoms of depression, independently of the effects of individual socio-economic and demographic characteristics (Ross 2000). Similarly, in recent studies, *neighbourhood* income has been significantly related to the prevalence of diagnosed schizophrenia and of substance abuse (Goldsmith, Holzer and Manderschied 1998). Independently of personal characteristics, such as sex and socio-economic opportunities, poorer neighbourhoods have been shown to provide fewer 'opportunity structures' for health-promoting activities than more affluent ones (Ellaway *et al.* 1997). Such studies underline the importance of distinguishing between individual-defined and neighbourhood-defined social position as sources of psychological stress and experienced distress.

The interaction between people and places

The interaction of 'people and places' has become increasingly important within models of physical health inequalities (Wilkinson *et al.* 1998) and concepts associated with 'neighbourhood' have relevance for tracking influences on mental health and understanding social divisions (e.g., Curtis and Rees-Jones 1998; McIntyre *et al.* 1993). These include: the physical features of the environment; the availability and quality of local health and welfare services; and the social and cultural features of neighbourhoods. The political, economic, ethnic and religious histories of localities vary, as do the extent of community integration, locally perceived threats to safety and particular neighbourhood reputations (McIntyre *et al.* 1993).

The constructs of 'locale' and 'cultural landscape', which attempt to provide a dynamic, multifactorial ecological frame for individual experience and action, have been used to situate health and health-related behaviour in specific places. 'Locale' has been deployed as an analytical device for understanding the way in which key social agents and programme agencies aspire to mobilise and produce positive effects in the context of changes in urban and rural areas (Duncan and Savage 1989). 'Cultural landscape' refers to the health-creating or health-damaging effects emanating from a combination of subjective and environmental influences in a particular place (Curtis and Rees-Jones 1998; Gesler 1992). An advantage of such theorising is that it counteracts the tendency mentioned previously to treat the socio-economic status of individuals as a simple proxy for the contexts in which they live (Dohrenwend 2000).

In a number of studies, additional effects, over and above a relationship with individual SES, have been ascribed to people living in poor neighbourhoods. Compared to similar individuals, defined by SES, in affluent areas, those in poor environments: achieve lower levels of education and economic success; engage in more criminal acts; and become victims of violence and crime more frequently (Silver 2000; South and Crowder 1997). Similarly, the distribution of housing stressors (e.g., overcrowding and dampness), together with perceptions of the local environment (area reputation), in part, explain the relationship between housing tenure and both physical and mental health (Ellaway and Macintyre 1998). Macintyre and her colleagues have shown that psychological characteristics are distributed unequally across several categories, in ways which are likely to have health impacts on those who rent property compared to owner-occupiers. The latter have been shown to have greater mastery, self-esteem and overall life satisfaction than those who rent (Macintyre *et al.* 1993).

Multiple locality stressors and resources which are potential protective factors, such as community housing support and primary care, have been shown to interact to produce particular local influences on the mental health of residents. Elliott (2000) has commented:

> Neighbourhood stressors and resources may increase individual vulnerability to stress by reducing the effectiveness of individual resources, such as when the combination of rampant crime and scarce police protection render neighbourhood residents impotent against larger forces, regardless of their personal sense of control. (Elliott 2000)

A study of Wythenshawe, an inner-city area of Manchester found that higher symptoms scores are associated with less neighbourliness/security, fewer leisure opportunities and a sense reported by residents that their area is in decline (Huxley *et al*. 2001). This type of study points to the way in which neighbourhoods themselves vary in the ratio of stressors and buffer resources impacting on stress levels, over and above those considered in traditional SES studies of mental health.

This focus on 'neighbourhood' as a transactional setting, in these and other studies, takes us beyond a traditional epidemiological approach, which, as we have argued earlier, has a tendency to prioritise compositional over contextual effects.[1] Whilst residents of poor localities tend to be poor themselves, contextual factors affecting mental health in neighbourhoods illuminate processes relevant to gender and race as well as social class (Elliott *et al*. 1996; Sampson *et al*. 1997; Silver *et al*. 1999).

An example of this point is provided by Schwabe and Kodras (2000), who investigated the propensity towards psychological distress across four US communities, using a qualitative study of local conditions. In their study, racialised features were found to vary substantially across the four sites. One area, which had a higher propensity towards distress amongst low SES black people, relative to their white counterparts, was linked by the researchers to the historical background of race relations in the locality. It had 'a relatively small, poor, less educated black population, recently drawn into lower-end jobs and finding little political expression, living in a distinctly disadvantaged position in this New England town'. The researchers then point to two distinctive aspects of New Haven, which were important in explaining differential mental health status:

First, the disparity between the prospects of this black population and lives of America's intellectual elite, living in immediate proximity, is particularly visible. Second, race differentials are striking *within* the lower socio-economic group, as white working class ethnic groups have dominated local politics, giving a greater sense of control over life chances. (Schwabe and Kodras 2000: 251)

The researchers concluded that the evident racial disparities in economic opportunities and political power, in New Haven, meant that the pressures and tensions, accompanying the disadvantaged position of low SES black people, would be reflected in a greater propensity towards psychological distress (Schwabe and Kodras 2000).

The impact of social disorganisation

The 'ambient hazards' of chaotic localities have been associated with an increase in depression, anxiety and behaviour disorders (Aneshensel and Succoff 1996). People living in 'socially disorganised' localities are more likely to experience psychological distress because of exposure to uncontrollable life events and psychosocial insults (Silver *et al.* 1999), and are more likely than others to be affected negatively by stressful life events, such as unemployment, family disruption, violence and crime, and to have fewer supportive relationships. A speedy turnover of local residents means the loss of existing relationships and it inhibits the establishment and maintenance of social ties (Sampson 1988). Social disorganisation decreases social integration,[2] which in turn increases the likelihood that individuals exist in a state of social isolation. This lack of social cohesion subsequently leads to a propensity to mental health problems.

The way in which contextual effects, such as social disorganisation, may interact with the experience of other individual aspects of disadvantage provides a means of understanding the relationship between external environment and feelings of psychosocial well-being. There is some evidence that the contextual effects of neighbourhood disadvantage on adult psychological well-being are mediated by people's perceptions of the locality as a chaotic and threatening place and the means that people perceive themselves to have in managing or dealing with external threats.

Our argument about the relevance of lay knowledge to understanding inequalities is relevant here and, in particular, the connections people themselves make between the social environment and mental health status. We have shown in our previous work how lay people hold on to a social causation view about mental health problems, whilst at the same time being aware that personal agency is the main tenable means of dealing with daily threats to psychological well-being (Rogers and Pilgrim 1997). Such lay knowledge can also be fruitfully linked to understanding the influences of neighbourhood character on mental health as a means of understanding the full personal and social picture. An analysis of Community Crime and Health Data of Illinois residents found that people who reported living in neighbourhoods with high levels of crime, vandalism, graffiti, danger, noise and drugs were more 'mistrusting'. According to the authors of this study, the powerlessness which ensued amplified the effect of neighbourhood disorder on mistrust (Ross, Mirowsky and Pribesh 2001).

Using multi-level data to explore the neighbourhood disadvantage effects on adult depression, Ross recently concluded that 'the breakdown of social control and order in one's neighbourhood is the major link between neighbourhood disadvantage and individual levels of depression' (Ross 2000: 184). The nuances of such a link in a different cultural context are illuminated by a recent qualitative study undertaken by one of us (AR) with colleagues[3] in the UK of Wythenshawe, an inner-city area of Manchester (Huxley *et al.* 2001). In-depth interviews with residents indicated how the perceived failure of external agencies responsible for urban regeneration and social control policies leads to an amplification of threat and a reliance on individualised coping strategies to tackle social nuisance which enhance a sense of entrapment.

Narrative accounts from respondents illuminated the way in which locality influenced key determinants of psychological well-being, such as 'restricted opportunities' and 'life events'. With regard to the latter, one man's depressed mental health state, which he attributed to the loss of his job, had abated after a year. Long-established networks and familiarity with the neighbourhood had seemingly played a role in his recovery. For other respondents, it was clear that the stresses of the urban locality had not only led to proximate psychological outcomes, such as panic attacks following harassment by 'out of control' teenagers in the vicinity, but had also provoked longer-term changes in lifestyle that fed into a restriction of his opportunities and the lowering of his personal goals.

Blocked or absent personal goals are consistently associated with poor mental health outcomes, as illustrated by these quotes from two middle-aged women living on the estate. This middle-aged woman described how she curtails individual efforts to improve her living arrangements and personal goal-setting as a response to vandalism and petty theft from her garden by young people:

> It annoys you. It annoys you. You think you try and make places look nice and you've got to come home to this. You know when you come home from wherever you've been and you come home to that. It's like all the stuff out of the garden that went. You don't feel as though you want to put any more into it. You want to buy things and you think 'why should I spend that', when it's, you know, you're working hard for it and you go out and that's gone and this has gone.

In the second account, benefits from work are under threat in her neighbourhood:

> With the new job I've got, in six months time I will be entitled to a brand new car, all expenses paid except for petrol and I am frightened to take it. How can I live with it? They said 'well don't worry it is all insured and taxed and that', but I said 'but what if every five minutes I am claiming for the car? Will it get taken off me? What's going to happen?' So I'm frightened. I keep saying 'no'. I don't think I will have the car. So I'm losing out, that's part of my salary. So I'm losing that now because I'm too scared to have a car upon my drive.

The analysis just presented points to the extent to which various locality initiatives designed to address inequalities are able to increase or diminish feelings of security and control. These are increasingly being seen as important by policy makers in addressing materialist and structural resources which contribute to dimensions of disadvantage. In this regard, a key construct, which focuses attention on collective and contextual resources in bringing about improvements in socially disadvantaged areas, is that of 'social capital'. This latter term has been defined as 'the features of social organisations, such as civic participation, norms of reciprocity, and trust in others, that facilitate co-operation for mutual benefit' (Kawachi *et al.* 1997 1491). We turn to the relevance that this has recently assumed for reversing area-based social exclusion later when discussing the policy context of social rejection.

Before that, given that neighbourhood conditions seem to be vital to our understanding of the genesis of 'common mental health problems' such as anxiety and depression, we turn to their impact on psychiatric patients with a diagnosis of severe mental illness.

The spatial distribution of deviant populations

The concentration of people with mental health problems in large asylums, located on the urban fringes during the nineteenth century, provided a reference point for analysing or advocating community care policies during the twentieth century and for understanding the status of the insane within a wider social order. The programme of hospital closure focused public and academic attention on the old 'asylum' and its excluding function for a wider community ('out of sight and out of mind').

In its favour, the asylum system provided local communities with employment and stability in times of economic and social turbulence. It also offered some opportunity for social mobility for those occupying lower social class positions. Those who harboured reservations about the demise of the asylum system represented it as a humane and homely place compared to the alternatives such as prison. However, its critics emphasised the contrast between inhumane total institutions and community living, with its enabling and supportive *gemeinschaft* qualities. For the mental health users' movement, in particular, the asylum symbolised oppression, whilst its demise offered the prospect of liberation and a new civil status (Rogers and Pilgrim 1991). As we note in Chapter 6, in relation to Russell Barton's work on institutional neurosis, the legacy of the Second World War and the Nazi concentration camps ensured that Western democracies would become sensitive about segregating devalued populations.

For some time after the advent of deinstitutionalisation policies the progress with community care policies could be evaluated by examining whether or not patients remained socially excluded. The implementation of Law 180 in Italy, for example, illuminated the radical agenda of some service providers compared to others. There was, to a large extent, a reliance on local product champions and adherence in localities to a radical mental health agenda of inclusion and civil rights of previously incarcerated patients. The emergence of dynamic and enlightened services in South Verona, for example, contrasted with other areas with apparently similar demographies and locality profiles. Notwithstanding such examples, postinstitutional images of 'the community' and locality-based patterns of attendant service provision have not been as easy to characterise or caricature as the old hospitals. This, in turn, is likely to impact on the ability to portray or map the extent of the needs of those with mental health problems and how they are met, or to assess and identify the nature and levels of experienced exclusions. However, the spatial segregation of people with mental health problems in adverse community settings, such as the inner city, has been a focus of critical attention, even for those, such as Andrew Scull, who offered a sustained critique of the asylum system:

> the alternative to the institution has been to be herded into newly emerging 'deviant ghettoes', sewers of human misery and which is conventionally defined as social pathology within which (largely hidden from outside inspection or even notice) society's refuse may be repressively tolerated. (Scull 1977: 153)

Whereas neo-Marxian critics like Scull emphasised the economic basis for the devaluation of people with mental health problems, in and out of hospital, more conservative critics adopted a victim-blaming approach, suggesting that people with disabling psychiatric conditions self-select or choose to live in poor neighbourhoods or become homeless (see Chapter 5). Medical studies of police referrals to psychiatric institutions, for example, tended to stress an isolated population from socially disorganised areas who drift into the inner city. Yet empirical studies of psychiatric referrals from the police suggest that most people come from, and are housed in, the locality rather than having 'drifted' in from outside the area (Rogers 1990).

The importance of the 'spatial' in analysing social marginalisation has been highlighted by studies showing an increasing concentration of community facilities and mental health workers in areas with high numbers of ex-psychiatric patients ('ghettoisation') and their exclusion from affluent areas (Dear and Wolch 1987; Sayce 2000; Wallace and Wallace 1997). A number of studies, mainly from the USA, suggested that day centres were springing up in close proximity to one another and these were near to specialised residential facilities, such as group homes and other forms of sheltered accommodation. This meant that psychiatric patients, and others using community services, were coming to characterise particular localities. These so-called 'service-dependent' ghettos were inner-city localities whose character was dominated by health and welfare services being targeted on the poorest residents (Dear and Wolch 1987).

This North American picture did not obtain in Britain immediately following hospital rundown. In the UK, at least as far as the early discharge of psychiatric patients was concerned, the relocation of patients from the first closing asylums was subject to careful planning . However, to an extent, a process of trans-institutionalisation is now evident, which has acted to conceal and segregate people within distinct geographical areas (Carpenter 2000), although these are configured differently according to the way in which national health care systems are funded. According to Carpenter, in Britain, the old hospitals have been largely replaced by 'a medically dominated "downsized" public psychiatric system, giving increasing priority to the treatment and containment of seriously disordered users, partly pressured by public concerns about risk and dangerousness' (Carpenter 2000).

Social rejection in its community and policy context

In the immediate aftermath of the early deinstitutionalisation programmes in the US and UK, research tended to concentrate on readmission as a signifier of success or failure in the adjustment of psychiatric patients to community living. Initially, then, there was little focus on how patients operated within the community contexts they found themselves in, how they managed with everyday living or the adversities they encountered. Subsequently, some researchers concerned with the social position and conditions of postinstitutionalised living for ex-psychiatric patients turned their attention to exploring the contextual factors which acted as a link between social and personal factors and social structure/formation (e.g., Dear and Laws 1986; Estroff 1981; Giggs 1987).

Labelling and stigma and its impact in community settings were found to be mediated by social-psychological processes of self-esteem and the negative self-concept which many psychiatric patients carry from a combination of their primary disability and from the cumulative reactions of others. Social rejection is an ongoing experience in community settings and a persistent form of social stress for discharged patients. Experiences of social rejection increase feelings of self-deprecation, which act to weaken a sense of mastery and self-control (Barham and Haywood 1991).

These experiences are evidence of consistent prejudice and discrimination (leading some in the mental health service users' movement to use the term 'mentalism' as an analogue to racism). The receipt of anti-psychotic medication has been found to be linked to the internalisation by patients of norms about the coercive consequence of non-compliance and a sense of gratitude for being 'allowed' to live in the community (Rogers *et al.* 1998). Estroffs' (1981) ethnographic study showed how the expectation and avoidance of stigma led to restricted social networks of ex-psychiatric patients. More recently, a longitudinal study found that exposure to stigmatising experiences from postinstitutional living (e.g., negative or avoidance attitudes from others) constitutes a source of serious and recurrent stress. In turn, this has the effect of reducing feelings of self-mastery and has long-term implications for a person's ability to function fully in society (Wright *et al.* 2000). As well as this study, which provided support for modified labelling theory,[4] another study has shown, from service users' own accounts, that rehabilitation pathways to 'independent living' are characterised by users feeling under pressure to live an ordinary life. As a result, many users' lives are characterised by socio-spatial isolation, large periods spent alone, restricted social networks and small activity spaces.

'Safe havens' (such as friends' houses and pubs) characterise the postinstitutional worlds of many ex-patients, rather than acceptance and inclusion by wider community networks and support systems (Pinfold 2000). Whilst some models of service provision (such as Assertive Community Treatment) include a focus on managing the impact of stigma on individuals, the wide-scale adoption of 'brokerage' models of mental health work have not emerged (at least in the UK). Other research has suggested that contact with community services fails to mitigate, in a significant way, such a sense of poor self-worth, as indicated by Wright *et al.* (2000) when discussing the results of their research on social rejection:

> Traditional forms of community-based care (i.e., group homes, partial hospitalisation and vocational rehabilitation) often touted by mental

health reformers as a potential solution for the negative effects of institutionalisation, appear to have only modest and short-lived effects on our
respondents' feelings of mastery and indirectly their self-esteem. (Wright
et al. 2000: 80)

There are suggestions, though, that access to social support from
friendship and benign familial networks can improve the self-worth
of psychiatric patients (Pescosolido *et al.* 1998). This implies that
'humane neighbourhoods', which include the social support mechanisms through which patients support one another, can act to reverse
social exclusion. This notion provides a link with the discussion of
contextual and compositional aspects of neighbourhood implicated
in the genesis of psychological problems discussed above.

The introduction of locality-based initiatives in areas of social
deprivation begs questions about how changes in environment are
likely to improve, or detrimentally affect, mental health over time.
For example, how might such policy initiatives interact with, and
impact upon, pre-existing social arrangements, networks norms and
values within a particular locality? What are the specific mechanisms
which might link the properties of a neighbourhood to the mental
health of its residents?

Spatial redistribution of the threat of risk and danger

A further dimension of social exclusion relates to people with
a mental health problem being seen as a source of risk and danger.
In the UK during the 1990s, first a Conservative and then a Labour
administration emphasised risk management in their mental health
policies. Such a focus had been evident in other cultural contexts
(Dallaire *et al.* 2000). Given that the great majority of psychiatric
patients are not dangerous (see Chapter 6), this risk emphasis has
skewed official appraisals of community care. For example, the mental health policy messages from the 1997–2001 Labour Government
were that community care had failed; psychiatric patients were a
danger or a nuisance; dedicated units were needed for the preventive
detention of personality disordered patients; and new legal powers
were required to enforce treatment in the community (Rogers and
Pilgrim 2001).

With regard to the issue of the management of risk, recent mental
health policy has, to a large extent, through 'transinstitutionalisation'

and a customary distrust of madness, invented new legal measures (such as compulsory outpatient treatment). This seems to be an attempt to recapture the security associated with the bygone age of total confinement. State-funded services are viewed as needing to provide the function of the old asylums within circumscribed community spaces in order to produce a 'system in which patient, carer and the public are safe and where security and support are provided to all who need it ... more acute mental health beds, more hostels and supported accommodation' (DoH 1998a). Such policy emphasis acts to reinforce the social exclusion of people with mental health problems by raising the salience of their risk and paying poor attention to their civil rights or their citizenship.

In addition to these policy inspired messages to view psychiatric patients with a certain degree of distrust, the latter also must contend frequently with poverty and neighbourhood animosity. The self-identity of the psychiatric patient is a persistent, rather than transient, state which is elaborated upon in locality contexts where stigma and derision exist. Some evidence suggests that conservative middle-class communities are most likely to exhibit extreme negative reactions to discharged mental patients, which have a deleterious impact on the social integration and morale of people in local communities. Liberal, non-traditional neighbourhoods conform most closely to the ideal accepting community (Segal *et al.* 1980).

Locality-based mental health policy

There is both a broad and more specific policy context for situating this complex picture of locality influences on mental health. Recent health policies emphasising the need to tackle health inequalities and promote population health have been accompanied by a greater awareness of the importance of local environments in the understanding of the origins of disorder and as a locus for intervention. In turn, these have been closely linked to urban regeneration policies.

In the UK, urban regeneration packages have been established since the late 1960s. These have encompassed a number of strands which relate to improving various economic, social and physical elements of local environments. One of the recent developments in urban regeneration has been the establishment of the Single Regeneration Budget Challenge Fund (SRB), introduced in 1994 and administered via Government Regional Offices. The SRB combines twenty formerly separate programmes, from five government departments, into a single budget available to provide more flexible funding for local regeneration. The allocation of resources for SRB programmes is now in its sixth annual round and responsibility for the programme has passed from the Department of Environment, Transport and the Regions (DETR) to the newly established Regional Development Agencies in England. In theory, this approach offers greater integration than previous programmes of British urban regeneration.

There is evidence of a more holistic approach within this type of regeneration strategy. For example, SRBs are being implemented at a time when there are parallel initiatives designed to provide a 'joined up' approach to social and health needs. These have characterised recent government initiatives in specific areas of health and welfare and have included policies explicitly designed to reduce inequalities in health and social exclusion. These include: HAZs (health action zones); Healthy Living Centres; EAZs (education action zones); and Sure Start (to provide parenting support aimed at pre-school children). A major new area-based initiative ('New Deal for Communities') has been introduced by the DETR. In addition, a variety of specific area-based interventions have begun to be developed by a range of individual government departments (such as Department for Education and Employment, the Home Office, Cabinet Office, Lord Chancellor's Department, as well as the DETR). An important feature of this new generation of policy initiatives is the extent to which this approach will succeed in the aim of improving local areas more than the previous fragmented approach. Given that the determinants and influences on mental health are multi-causal, these social policy initiatives together form the bases upon which it is possible to provide locally tailored, multi-domain packages of risk reduction measures.

A number of small studies suggests that the risks associated with common mental health problems can be reduced by interventions targeted at those who have experienced job loss and unemployment (Price *et al.* 1992; Vinokur *et al.* 1991) and teenage pregnancy in the context of poverty (Olds *et al.* 1988). There is also some indication that the mental health of the population can be raised by improvements to housing and the local area by reducing the 'ambient hazards' we noted earlier (Halpern 1980). For example, rehousing on the grounds of mental health has been shown to impact positively on anxiety and depression (Elton and Packer 1986).

A range of employment initiatives has been created in Europe during the 1980s and 1990s as part of anti-poverty programmes which have potential benefits for mental health. These initiatives, which include a network of work cooperatives operating in Germany, Ireland, Italy and Switzerland, have provided opportunities for promoting self-esteem and self-management and a positive strategy for addressing marginalisation (Ramon 1996; Savio and Righetti 1993). Financial resources and the reconstruction of housing have been found to make a critical difference to recovery from mental health crises which arise from major disruption in or destruction of people's living environments (Wang *et al.* 2000). However, policy initiatives, such as urban regeneration, have been introduced in a context in which there is little government understanding of the way in which changes in the socio-economic circumstances of a community affect the mental health and quality of life of citizens. There has been an increasing resort to the notion of social capital as a means of filling this gap.

Amelioration through social capital?

Whereas 'social disorganisation' is indicative of poor mental health, 'social capital' is ameliorative in its emphasis. Social capital refers to the combined resources of individuals and their integration into expressed local communal activity – sporting, religious, educational, cultural and artistic events and routines. It is described by Portes (1998) as: 'the ability to secure benefits through membership in networks and other social structures'. Theoretically, with increased social capital comes increased emotional well-being in those participating and in those simply residing nearby. With parochial collective activity come social ties, mutual welfare, civic pride and public friendliness. In areas with low social capital, these features of local life are either sparse or absent.

Given these positive attributed features of social capital, it has begun to make a contribution to the understanding of social disadvantage, alongside more traditional variables such as social class or SES. Also, from a social policy perspective, social capital has a potential for pointing up means of ameliorating social ills and in promoting and sustaining mentally healthy local communities and is increasingly offered as a strategy for community- and capacity-building (Hawe and Shiell 2000). The link between social capital and psychological well-being has been associated with 'opportunity structures', such as social support networks which enhance the self-esteem and self-efficacy of their participants (Lomas 1998). Thus, in ecological terms, 'collective efficacy' – the actions and willingness of local residents to participate in community activities – has been associated with changes in rates of health-related behaviour across different neighbourhoods (Sampson *et al.* 1997). Additionally, the relational properties of social networks operating at a microlevel are considered to be important for understanding the genesis of mental health problems and for promoting mental health. According to Woolcock (1998) 'the more intensive the social ties and generalized trust within a given community, the higher its "endowment" of social capital'.

Policy makers in Germany, the UK and the USA have shown an intense interest in the notion of social capital as a means of addressing the problems associated with disorganised communities. However, others have been sceptical of the undue reliance placed on this as a means of addressing locality inequalities because of the way in which it is seemingly being portrayed and deployed as an alternative to improved material resources and more equitable social structures. Muntaner *et al.* (2000) for example sum up objections, namely:

> It presents itself as an alternative to materialist structural inequalities (class, gender and race) and invokes a romanticised view of communities without social conflict... social capital is used in public health as an alternative to both state-centred economic redistribution and party politics, and represents a potential privatization of both economics and politics.

The restricted networks, social rejection and stigma which seem resilient to the existing efforts of community rehabilitative services for those with mental health problems suggests that those with long-term mental health problems are currently unlikely to be participants or beneficiaries of social capital initiatives.

Mental health policy has been characterised by paradoxical imperatives. On the one hand, as we noted earlier, there has been an emphasis on the prejudicial and authoritarian management of the perceived risk that those with a mental health problem are deemed to pose (principally) to others. On the other hand, there is a whole raft of policies directed at the amelioration of social exclusion. In the first of these, the 'community', as a social space, is seen as an arena in which the public have been placed at risk through the abandoning of the old policy of segregation. The focus here has been on greater coercive control. The second countervailing imperative is a commitment to addressing the social marginalisation and exclusion of poor and vulnerable groups. Here, there is an interest in destigmatisation, the social conditions that give rise to, or exacerbate, distress and dysfunction.

The focus on risk (which we discussed earlier) has meant that governments have progressed with reforms encouraging the use of compulsion and surveillance which are seemingly influenced by public fears and a media-fuelled link between dangerousness and mental health. With regards to reversing social exclusion, an alternative set of responses is propounded. Mental health sits alongside other areas of quality improvements in the health and social welfare agenda and is tied to policies designed to address urban and community problems as a means of promoting social inclusiveness.

For example, the National Service Framework for Mental Health (NSF), which represents part of a wider Clinical Governance (quality) agenda[5] in the UK, connects mental health to social inclusion. Standard 1 of the NSF is designed to ensure Health and Social Services promote mental health and reduce the discrimination and social exclusion associated with mental health problems. Here, an individual emphasis on engendering emotional resilience is paralleled by a focus on social capital, citizenship and programmes about community improvement (DoH 1999).

Divergent policy strictures pose a dilemma as far as tackling mental health inequalities are concerned. In particular, the paradoxical policy imperatives and language of official mental health policy, which is no longer bounded solely to the role of mental hospital, brings about a new social division. A conceptual split in this policy formation and implementation is forced between those who are precariously distressed (to be empathised with) and an alien category of disordered person who poses a serious and unpredictable threat to others living in the community to be distrusted. With regard to the first of these, urban and social policy initiatives may do much to tip the balance in favour of those who are precariously distressed by reducing levels of psychological stress in community populations. However, this is likely to contrast negatively with new mechanisms of control and containment for those who would previously have been contained behind hospital walls and are still viewed as a distinct alien category.

Conclusion

'Neighbourhood' has been associated in complex ways with mental health and inequalities. This is because the stress of adverse social environments can contribute directly to psychological distress and dysfunction, and because local contexts are crucial in establishing norms of acceptance or rejection for those with mental health problems living in 'open settings'. The analysis of locality influences points to the diffuse and varied ways in which they can produce or mitigate mental health problems and social inequalities. Resources, such as social capital, entail a form of psychosocial rather than economic wealth – the ability and opportunity to be involved in community networks and activities. As with economic wealth, it can be present in abundance or it can be depleted, with predictable consequences.

Social capital and mental health are mutually reinforcing. Levels of depression, linked as they are to social and material resources, are not only indicative of the levels of relative deprivation in a community. They are also likely to impact on the ability of local populations to mobilise, or take advantage of, resources of change. Low-grade depression amongst a significant number of people in a community is likely to inhibit such activity. Recent British social policy is playing a paradoxical role by promoting social inclusion in impoverished neighbourhoods, whilst at the same time fostering the social exclusion of people with mental health problems by contributing to them being stereotyped as dangerous. More will be noted about the importance of local 'ambient hazards' in Chapter 5. The extent to which the policy emphasis on dangerousness is warranted will be addressed in Chapter 6.

A final point to note about the relationship and context of neighbourhood with mental health is the enduring schism between transinstitutionalised service provision and other parts of everyday social, personal and economic life. The connectedness between the spheres of service provision (provided, for example, in local out-patient departments or acute district general hospital psychiatric units) and the economic and social life of the community increasingly occupies a similar geographical space. However, the sharing of social space does not equate with models that connect the two spheres despite a rhetoric from mainstream psychiatric epidemiology that suggests that representative information in a defined geographical area can estimate the extent of unmet needs and the services required to meet those needs (Jenkins 2001).

In reality, the service models deployed by most contemporary mental health services to meet mental health needs that arise in localities remain as remote from one another as the geographical boundaries which demarcated the Victorian asylums from the outside world. Thus, whilst, for example, the causes of young male suicide may be seen as emanating from the social conditions of disadvantaged localities and hospitals are designated with the reduction of risk, a policy response that is effective in managing risk and ameliorating the social causes of such a problem across both services and non-service arenas remains elusive. In this respect, the failure to develop effective locality-based responses from services that coalesce with the broader social context represents a major hurdle to tackling social inequalities. As we explore in the next two chapters, professional and service responses remain cut off from the processes generated in broader society related to mental health in other ways.

3

Inequalities created by service provision

Introduction

Service provision may cause, aggravate or ameliorate mental health problems. Broadly, mental health professionals (with some notable exceptions) have tended to emphasise only the ameliorative role of services. Moreover, politicians and lay people may assume that service contact is unambiguously positive. Consequently, equality of access is simply taken to be a desirable political goal. By contrast, critical commentators and disaffected service users have tended to critique professional services for their iatrogenic impact. The dehumanising impact of the mental asylum on the lives of its inmates formed a sociological focus in the 1950s and 1960s that illuminated the social divisions that demarcated the mental patient from the rest of society. Some critical psychiatrists sought to reverse this picture by addressing the injuries of adverse social and personal circumstances that arose from contact with mental institutions. For example, some existential and psychoanalytical psychiatrists responded to the latter by trying to humanise services with the introduction of experimental therapeutic communities.

The notion of separation or sequestration of some people from wider society is reflected in the comparators used by Erving Goffman in his notion of 'total institutions' – monasteries, prisons and concentration camps – which contained those who, by definition, are 'different' from those residing in open settings. As a result of this physical separation, the social injuries of those with mental health problems have, with a few exceptions, been relatively divorced from other disadvantaged population groups. 'Progress' for people with mental health problems has thus been associated with improved organisational arrangements. For example, the philosophy of normalisation sought to reverse the impact of secondary deviance caused by mental illness and mental handicap hospitals. Thus, the psychological and physical impact of the total institution is a constant source of reference for these critical and oppositional strategies. By contrast, improving the lot of other disadvantaged groups in 'open society' has been judged more by other criteria, such as enhanced income maintenance or access to educational opportunities, transport, etc.

Lessons from the institution

Given the centrality of the Victorian institution to social policy and to subsequent critiques of the management of madness, a number of points can be noted in relation to social divisions and mental health. Originally, the large institutions contained ideas of social betterment. Moral treatment was essentially an attempt to recover madness from its alien state and bring it back within the moral order of wider society. However, the ideals of moral treatment, and with it notions of equity and the social improvement of inmates, was abandoned almost immediately. There is some evidence that inmates of asylums sometimes were sheltered from the consequences of adverse social and financial circumstances (e.g., the Great Depression of the 1930s) (Gittens 1998), thus conferring an advantage compared to the sane poor. However, in overall terms, the impact of institutionalisation was overwhelmingly one of social rejection, stigmatisation and even demonisation. A variety of studies of institutional life exposed the social disability and disadvantage created by an inpatient status (Barton 1958; Brown and Wing 1962; Goffman 1961; Rosenhan 1973). This body of empirical work focused on the design of the mental institution and the impact of such arrangements on the identity of the individual and the formation of 'secondary deviance'. Inpatients were subjected to numerous 'assaults on the self'. The routines of institutional life (e.g., the 'degradation ceremony' of taking possessions and personal clothing away) stripped people of their external sense of self or identity and had a demoralising and dehumanising impact on the individual. The 'mortification of the self' and role dispossession illuminated a great division between the sane and insane. The admitted patients lost their sense of personal safety and individuality. Social contact was both controlled and enforced by staff. Day-to-day life was regulated by professionally defined rules and the residential milieu could be oppressive or benign at the whim of staff discretion.

John Martin's book, *Hospitals In Trouble* (1985), attributed a series of scandals about neglect and abuse in British mental institutions, between 1965 and 1983, to a 'corruption of care' fostered by concomitant layers of isolation (e.g., geographical, personal and professional). However, because isolation was inherent to institutions (they were designed *to be* isolated), the notion of their humane reform became ultimately problematic. Also, Martin's notion of the 'corruption of care' reflected the paternalism intrinsic to mental health work. 'Corruption' indicates paternalism gone astray.

The total institution had a near totalising effect on any academic critique of the social inequalities associated with the role of mental patient. Goffman, Martin and others remained focused on the institution as the primary source of injustice for those with mental health problems. This inadvertently obscured factors external to the asylum and blocked a deeper analysis of the social exclusion of people with mental health problems emerging. Rather, attention focused on ways of reforming or aboloshing these organisations.

Given the problem of the institution, the first practical attempt at its reform entailed a rediscovery of the tenets of moral treatment. Therapeutic communities (TCs) were designed to make the social environment of hospital life the main therapeutic tool. They were pioneered in Britain during the Second World War by psychotherapeutically oriented psychiatrists. The practical pressure for this was the sheer numbers of military psychiatric casualties. Individual therapy was unfeasible and so small- and large-group work was invented, with the ward being reframed as a 'community'.

Whilst the philosophies behind TCs emerged from differing psychiatric positions, they shared a vision of the social structure of the ward, with its atmosphere and morale being cast as elements in a synergistic therapeutic endeavour. For some more radical innovators, this was accompanied by alternative conceptions of mental illness. For example, symptoms were seen as being socially constructed and 'schizophrenia' was conceptualised as a voyage into 'inner space'. The latter implied a healing duty to support the voyager through their journey. This radical amplification of early TC principles was associated with British 'anti-psychiatry' and the work of David Cooper and Ronald Laing (Crossley 1998).

The centrality of everyday lived experience in the ideology of TCs gave it a potential for understanding the genesis of mental health problems in the social divisions of wider society. However, the origins of the TC movement were not mainly about those excluded from civil society but a response to the casualties of warfare. Also, the potential of the TCs to extend to other population groups was circumscribed by their fundamental flaws as viable organisations. TCs often coexisted in or alongside the large asylums without seemingly impacting on them. Later, when large hospitals disappeared, and a quick 'throughput' in smaller acute DGH (District General Hospital) units was emphasised, the systemic stability of long periods of residence no longer existed. These factors led to TCs being pushed to the margins of the British mental health industry. They are now specialised units (such as the Henderson in London and Webb House in Crewe) mainly dealing with people with a diagnosis of personality disorder. The history of TCs emphasised the relevance of communication and reflective democracy. This was deemed to be suited to those with neurotic or personality problems. Mainstream NHS psychiatry conceded this setup but did not see TCs as being suitable for psychotic patients.

The political aspirations of the British TC movement were an important but not sole stimulus for the emergence of Italian 'anti-psychiatry', which was more successful in linking external social conditions with the marginalisation of psychiatric patients in total institutions. A more holistic critique of psychiatry was evident in the work of Franco Basaglia, and the mental health reforms he championed in Italy placed social divisions centre-stage. In describing these reforms, Basaglia noted that they were 'More akin to the political struggles which broke out in other areas of social life in the 1960s breaking up established institutions and exposing their shortcomings, than to *avant-garde* psychiatric experiments like the therapeutic community in England or *la psychiatric institutionelle* in France' (Basaglia 1981: 185). The formation of *Psichiatria Democratica* was born of an alliance between trade unions, the students' movements and sections of the psychiatric profession. In particular, the trade unions were instrumental in linking the reform of psychiatric services with wider social and economic issues (Rogers and Pilgrim 1986). This connection, forged by the Italian reformers, between mental health and wider social injustice ensured the programmatic centrality of social inclusion, making this an Italian exception to a European rule.

In other countries, such as the UK, the lack of concern with the wider social context of people with mental health problems is, to a large extent, reproduced at the level of contemporary service provision. Despite the recognition of social isolation and the poverty of many patients, the wider agenda of social inclusion and access to employment remains marginal in mental health policy. Current models of case management in the UK have shown poor outcomes in terms of improving the quality of life of patients. The more intensive US equivalent PACT model (though not without its civil liberty controversies) includes intensive work outside psychiatric settings in the patient's own environment and employment context. It has shown better results in terms of fuller social integration and uptake of economic and social opportunities than standard case-management. However, despite the merits of this approach, policy-makers in the UK have remained reluctant to adopt the PACT model. The narrower administrative approach in the UK (the Care Programme Approach) has had the effect of separating a patient's treatment from their social context (although the views of relatives and significant others are included in the process).

Inequalities in mental health status versus inequalities in service provision

Most analyses of health problems and their management have focused *either* on epidemiology *or* on the management of illnesses within a service context. Services have traditionally been seen as having little to do with health status, save treatment having a tertiary prevention role of reducing the chances of relapse. To an extent, this split reflects divisions in the disciplinary organisation of health research. Medical and social epidemiologists, by and large, focus on aetiology or the social determinants of mental illness, whilst the newer discipline of health services research has been concerned with what happens inside services.

Recently, there have been some attempts to bridge the gap – particularly in relation to secondary prevention. Some public health debates have turned their attention to the relative contributions of access to services versus social determinants (Andrulis 1998). Socio-economically disadvantaged groups not only have greater needs but also have less access to help. As one of the authors (AR) and colleagues have argued elsewhere, greater attention needs to be paid to a 'whole systems' approach to access (Rogers *et al.* 1999), which links lay actions in the informal sector with the formal provision of care (and particularly primary care). Notwithstanding these newer developments, the connection between health status and health care delivery has been generally restricted to a matter of matching the supply of services with health needs.

Explanatory frameworks about the causes of mental health problems reinforce this divide by giving little consideration to *the impact* (rather than the availability) of service contact. The social causation thesis emphasises the social and environmental causes of a mental health problem. The social selection thesis suggests that mental health problems lead to social isolation, altered employment and housing opportunities and downward social mobility. Both of these competing explanatory frameworks ignore the evidence that service contact makes a contribution to the social situation of individuals. Hospitalisation can adversely disrupt an individual's personal and social situation (Bean and Mounser 1993). Mortality, particularly from suicide, increases in the period after a first admission to hospital (Appleby *et al.* 1999).

The paradox of the inverse care law in mental health policy

The inverse care law (ICL) is a foundational thesis which has shaped the analysis of inequalities in services provision. The ICL was described thirty years ago as 'the availability of good medical care tends to vary inversely with the need for it in the population served' (Tudor-Hart 1971). The 'law' is predicated on the notion that access to care has a tendency to increase with increasing class status, with the poorest people tending to get the poorest health care. This in turns leads to a situation in which those with the least need of health care use the health services more (and more effectively) than do those with the greatest need.

The ICL has constituted a dominant framework for understanding patterns of inequalities in health services and it has been clearly demonstrated in a number of areas. Such findings have been grist to the mill of vociferous arguments for increasing access to health services, including mental health care, for disadvantaged groups. Once there is evidence showing the unequal distribution of services relative to need, access to services becomes the political strategy considered most likely to ameliorate health disadvantage (Andrulis 1998).

There is a wealth of evidence indicating differences in the utilisation of mental health services by different groups in the population. In inpatient psychiatric services, as in some physical health services (e.g., cardiology), people from low social class backgrounds predominate (the reverse of the ICL). However, a range of evidence exists which supports the notion of an ICL operating in relation to mental health provision. Surveys of the use of primary care for mental health consultations of adults living in deprived multi-ethnic inner-city catchment areas have examined the association between clinical and demographic factors. These show that many people considered to have 'psychiatric morbidity' do not receive treatment either from primary care or specialist services (Commander *et al.* 1997a). Barriers seem to operate at particular points of the mental health service system and this varies for different groups in the population. For example, Commander *et al.* (1997b) identify an impediment to Asian people accessing care at the interface between primary and secondary care, whilst for Afro-Caribbean people 'the poor level of case recognition by GPs' may be responsible for poor uptake of services.

There is a tendency for such surveys about access to mental health services to be conducted without reference to the nature and purpose of the latter. As we noted in the introduction, a strong cultural tradition exists in which service provision is simply presumed to meet health need. The ICL framework is of limited utility when applied to mental health, basically because psychiatric services function in a substantially different way from other parts of the health service. We now turn to this difference.

The gradient of coercion operating in mental health services

Notwithstanding evidence for the variation in the quality of service provision, or for the clinical iatrogenesis created by modern health services, most interventions for physical health problems are voluntary and ameliorative in intent. By contrast, in psychiatric services lawful involuntary detention and treatment are explicit and prominent operational features. A proportion of patients are forcibly detained and treated by the use of therapeutic law; some are notionally voluntary but *de facto* detainees, and others are genuinely voluntary but exist in a service context where the threat of coercion is ever present. In the light of these peculiar features about psychiatry, mental health work can be conceptualised as part of a wider State apparatus which controls the social problems associated with poverty and the 'underclass' (Thomas and Romme 1997). Once conceived in this way, a unitary view of service contact as necessarily aiming for, or achieving, a gain in the mental health status of service recipients is rendered problematic.

The coercive role of psychiatry in response to certain types of social crisis and deviance has been a salient feature of sociological, historical and critical analysis of psychiatry (e.g., the work of Szasz, Laing, Scull and Goffman). Collectively, this body of work suggests that the function of psychiatry is different from other branches of medicine. In psychiatric services, the overrepresentation of people from a lower social class and some ethnic minorities in coercive contexts is not about meeting need in the same way that health services respond to physical problems.

Of course, not all service provision is coercive to the same degree. A graduated system of control operating in services is relevant to consider in making judgements about the extent to which services meet need. For example, some wards are locked in open psychiatric units ('intensive care units'). Some hospitals hold patients in conditions of 'medium security'. Others contain more dangerous mentally disordered offenders in high security conditions. However, the constant threat of repressive social control makes such a graduated system difficult to describe meaningfully by physical features alone.

Outside acute inpatient provision and forensic services, the coercive/social control function is lessened and the use of services is more akin to those for patients with physical conditions. However, even in primary care, the GP acts as a 'second' opinion medical practitioner in supporting applications for involuntary detention in hospital. This may mean that the possibility of compulsion and the stigma attached to secondary services may impact on the willingness to access and utilise primary care services (Rogers *et al.* 2001). Nevertheless, overall, primary care is less coercive than other parts of the mental health system. Primary care is the point in the State-run health care system which is principally influenced by patients' decision-making about when and how to access services. It is also the point where the social contract in providing a service free at the point of need is most meaningful, given the direct access that it permits to citizens. We discuss this in more detail in the next chapter.

The emergence of voluntary organisations, the increase of private practice and user-led services and self-management are significant changes in the pattern of service provision. The utilisation of non-State employees in the delivery of services also changes the nature of service delivery. The rise of self-employed primary care counsellors trained outside mainstream State-provided higher education for health professionals is an example here. In the US, users have taken on roles previously monopolised by mental health professionals. These user-led schemes have been noted for their greater success in providing less coercive services to people. Here, we consider a number of types of service in relation to coercion.

Inpatient services

The District General Hospital Unit (DGHU) was heralded as a less coercive and more community-oriented alternative to the old mental institutions. Assimilation with services for physically ill people by constructing services on the same site as general medical services was promoted by medical reformers as a vehicle for destigmatisation. Equating mental illness with physical illness has brought about a marginal integration at the level of knowledge. In its sophisticated form, 'liaison psychiatry' challenges the divorce between psyche and soma (e.g., in exploring conditions such as fibromyalgia and chronic fatigue syndrome). However, DGHU psychiatry has become increasingly coercive and non-therapeutic. Rates of admission have increased, especially for young men (Lelliott *et al.* 1996). Admissions are increasingly made under the Mental Health Act and overcrowding is rife. DGHUs are increasingly acting as a repository for people who are 'difficult' and cannot be managed by community services. These repositories are characterised by little recreational activity and little therapeutic input (Quirk and Lelliott 2001; Shepperd *et al.* 1997).

Private psychiatric services

The cash nexus and payment systems operating in the private sector suggests a relationship similar to private patients for physical illness.

Relationships are generally entered into voluntarily and the ability to pay negates the need to pass through various surveillance and justification mechanisms normally applied to NHS patients. This is clear in relation to accessing psychotherapy and other talking treatments. NHS rules, which are often implicitly applied, necessitate individuals having to meet certain criteria, and are not applicable in private services. These include the appropriateness to benefit from treatments and an assessment of patients' character and mental health career trajectory. These are frequently used in making judgements about the definition of and management of a mental health problem. Such professional judgements may not concur with those of the 'patient'. Residential private institutions operate within the rules laid down by mental health legislations and do, at times, resort to compulsory admissions or offer an overspill facility for 'extra-contractual referrals from the NHS'. However, it is common knowledge that people who can afford it (or their relatives) use these services as a means of avoiding the overt stigma and consequences that accrue from compulsory admission to NHS-run acute hospital wards.

Voluntary organisations

The balance between informal and formal service contact has implications for inclusion and exclusion. The therapeutic ethos of formally provided services is commonly promoted as a means of preventing deterioration and facilitating social inclusion. The need for formal services to engage with patients and prevent them from 'falling through the net' is increasingly embodied in the ethos of mental health service provision and in specific supportive legislation.

Leaving aside the effectiveness of specific actions, such as forced medication, as a means of effective social control, which does not purport to do anything about social divisiveness but is explicitly about issues to do with public and governmental perceptions of the best way in which to manage risk, the evidence for such contact having a socially inclusive role is equivocal. Whilst intensive case-management, or 'aggressive rehabilitation', can mediate the impact of stigma by enhancing peoples' sense of mastery, standard forms of community service seem to make little, if any, difference in this regard. A study of deinstitutionalisation and social rejection of patients from the US found that social rejection is a persistent source of social distress for discharged patients that weakens their sense of daily personal mastery (Wright *et al*. 2000)

> Where the patients received their follow-up care – whether in a commu-
> nity setting or in another state hospital – had little impact on their
> (patients) self-related feeling or on their experiences of social rejection
> (Wright *et al*. 2000: 68)

There is evidence that some users gain from service contact but in a different way from that assumed by specialists. A preference for GPs over psychiatrists is due to the use of lay knowledge and means of managing mental health problems that fit with the everyday notions of patients. Similarly, the most valued aspects of formally provided day provision are those things that are not provided on a professional basis; the social links and company of other users (Rogers and Pilgrim 1993). The reason for this discrepancy may be related to the professional action within State-regulated services which undermines client confidence. Professionals tend to block an ordinary identity and emphasise pathology, thus negating a client identity of a patient that is compatible with social inclusion and self-mastery. This point about professionally dominated services is illuminated here by Prior (1991) when describing practitioners' accounts of patients' activity:

> Once out of the client's hearing...the results of these interactions are
> often re-analysed in terms of a specific (and professionalised) linguistic
> framework. Thus a game of ten-pin bowling is re-analysed in terms of
> coping skills. A lapse of memory is discussed in terms of a syndrome and a
> leisure time activity is analysed in terms of affective disorder. In fact client
> 'problems' are in many respects newly created through the application of
> a behaviourist discourse into what are called 'activities of daily living'
> (Prior 1991: 141–2)

Structurally, the voluntary sector has a relatively distant relationship from statutorily provided services. Such services are characterised both by their popularity with users and their distance from traditional models of mental health service provision. Research conducted by us in the early 1990s showed that users who had used both statutory and non-statutory services were more positive about the voluntary sector. The reasons offered for this were related to the nature of the differing service provisions. Positive features of the voluntary sector included: informality; 'being treated as equals'; access to non-traditional interventions (e.g., self-help, mediating domestic/housing problems); mutuality and active engagement in providing services; and participation in local community life. These marked off users' experiences from those encountered in the statutory sector (Rogers *et al.* 1993).

Research reporting user preferences for voluntary services is confirmed by more orthodox evaluative methods. A recent randomised control trial found that people who were referred from primary care to a liaison organisation facilitating contact with voluntary organisations showed greater improvement compared with patients receiving routine general practitioner care. Those referred to the project had better mental health scores, found it easier to carry out everyday activities and had more positive feelings about general health and their quality of life than those who were not referred (Grant *et al.* 2000). The lack of formal responsibilities, especially for risk management, free up more opportunities for clients who use the voluntary sector.

User-provided services

One development of the service users' movement is the user-led service innovations. User-led services can be found in the voluntary sector in Britain, occasionally supported by statutory authorities. Mowbray *et al.* (1997) review the large range of user-controlled facilities available in the USA. This range of activity varies from the latent role of patients as self-caring and mutually supportive in professionally led services and self-help groups, right through to complex funded projects which are managed and staffed by users themselves (Chamberlin 1988; Lindow 1994). The type of service the latter provide (such as safe houses and drop-in day centres) reflect the users' movement's priorities of voluntary relationships, alternatives to hospital admission, crisis intervention and personal support.

Between the diffuse self-care strategies occurring spontaneously between patients in statutory services and funded user-led services, there is another layer of user involvement. In recent years, service providers have, to various degrees in different localities, sought the collaboration of users to support service developments. Minimally, this has entailed surveys or consultation exercises about local need identification (an extension of the role of user-as-consumer). It has also included: the formal acceptance by professional providers of innovations such as patients' councils; users being paid to train mental health staff (Crepaz-Keay *et al.* 1998) and users and 'carers' groups being called upon to improve services in collaborative experiments in service development (Carpenter and Sbaraini 1997; Pilgrim and Waldron 1998).

In the light of the above evidence of differentiated service use, professional activity and patient experience, there is a need to reappraise the relevance and applicability of the inverse care law to mental health service provision. The graduated system of social control and the divided loyalties of professionals evident in the latter render the ICL highly problematic as an analytical framework.

The relationship between need and supply

It is not only the nature and supply of service provision and the decision making of professionals in imposing services on individuals that are implicated in creating differential patterns of service provision. This represents only half the equation. The nature of service provision needs to be mapped against the type and expression of need and their associated mediating processes which connect need with service provision. The presence of coercion and the interests of significant others, we note above, extend to referral patterns and pathways into care.

Social networks and processes are a latent influence on help-seeking and service utilisation. In relation to physical health problems, the latter are generally seen as operating in a helpful or benign manner in connecting people with services. However, in the case of mental health service contact, these mediating processes, are more likely to arise from the needs of others, in particular the desire to control unwanted behaviour in identified patients. The 'betrayal funnel' discussed by Goffman describes a negative process of familial involvement in mediating psychiatric service contact. The way in which strangers respond to emotional deviance in public places is also implicated. A process of transmitted discrimination is evident in the response of the public to the behaviour of black people. For example, emergency police referrals to psychiatry are, in part, a conveyor belt for community prejudice, which appears in services and is recorded as 'mental health need' (Rogers 1990).

There is a range of complex and competing theories of need which we have discussed elsewhere (Pilgrim and Rogers 1999; Rogers and Pilgrim 2001). Here, we confine ourselves to discussing the nature of clinically defined, versus subjectively defined, need as these are the central notions around which demand for service provision revolve.

Different needs and their relationship to service provision

The notion of 'clinically defined need' retains its dominance in mental health services and definitions of mental health need in research and practice tend to use variables that conform to traditional psychiatric knowledge. As we have seen in the previous chapters, the clinical perspective is predicated either on an epidemiological or symptom-based definition (such as the level and type of symptom in the community) or on one defined by symptoms for which there is an 'effective' ameliorative or curative intervention.

Despite the rise in the popularity of eclectic definitions and port-manteau models, definitions of need based on psychiatric diagnosis continue to have the greatest salience. Indeed, even amongst disciplines adjacent to medicine, such as clinical psychology, which at times distance themselves from medically defined knowledge, psychiatric diagnostic criteria retain some popularity.

Another way in which service utilisation affects clinically defined need is via clinical concepts. This is clearly seen in relation to the somatisation thesis. From a traditional medical point of view, there is tendency to conceptualise Asian people as 'somatisers'. In the area of mental health, some psychiatric researchers suggest that Asian women in particular present their mental distress as bodily symptoms (Currer 1986). Somatisation has been described as the expression of personal and social distress in an idiom of bodily complaints with medical help-seeking. Such a conceptualisation is not only imbued with moral meaning, it also implicates professional value judgements about help-seeking and the use of services. According to Dworkin (1994), the two defining features of somatisation are the presence of numerous self-reported symptoms and 'excessive' help-seeking behaviour. The persistent presentation of physical symptoms in the absence of medically 'confirmed' organic pathology, together with increasing demand for medical care, are seen as imposing an increasing burden on the health service. The latter thinly disguises a medical view, which suggests that the expression of need in this way constitutes an unwarranted source of demand that should not be taken at face value.

There have been objections to the somatisation thesis and its associated medical moralisations. Fenton and Sadiq-Sangster (1996) point out that the presentation of bodily symptoms by Asian women is ambiguous for a number of reasons. They argue that it could mean several things:

(a) a non-recognition of mental illness, so that ailments are always presented as somatic,
(b) a non-recognition of the link between physical ailments and emotional states,
(c) a presentation of ailments as somatic despite some recognition of mental distress, and
(d) simply a non-presentation of mental symptoms to bio-medical doctors. (Fenton and Sadiq-Sangster 1996: 69).

This notion of 'somatised' mental health need has a number of implications for the provision and receipt of equitable care. For some practitioners, it provides a case for an apparently legitimate form of Western medical paternalism, that is, doctors need to diagnose and treat an underlying mental illness (depression) despite the patient's misguided somatic presentation. However, given the unexplored ambiguity noted above, the psychiatric assumption of somatisation in Asian populations is a pre-emptive construction.

The somatisation thesis has a tendency to stereotype whole groups of people and fails to incorporate reference to the situational contexts and meanings of the population groups. At the same time, it implies a precarious legitimacy in help-seeking. Generalisations are also made about other service provision. People may encounter different styles and qualities of mental health services in various parts of Britain. Despite this, the psychiatric literature studying differences in hospitalisation rates in Asian people assumes that these exist as a result of patient variables alone.

The main weaknesses of the clinical model are the marginalisation of subjective experience as a defining feature of mental health need and the utilisation of services. There might be a range of reasons why people are reluctant to disclose psychological distress, given the experience they have had with services. It is not unlikely that the 'somatisation' of symptoms is, in part, a function of the perception of primary care as a place which deals mainly with physical problems. From a patient perspective, this creates an ambivalence about contact with medical services as a means of solving the personal and social problems which lie behind 'depression'. In a cultural context of family loyalty and a need for privacy, this ambivalence may be more profound.

Need and personal identity

One consequence of the dominance of clinical notions of need is not only the marginalisation of need defined subjectively but also its manifestation within and consequences for service provision. Whilst some social science definitions do incorporate absolute notions of health need, which are not dissimilar from clinical perspectives (Doyal and Gough 1991), most emphasise the relative nature of need. This starts from the premise that an individual sufferer's needs may be constructed by the extent to which symptoms disrupt everyday activities and the extent to which they are fearful or embarrassing. This notion of need also highlights the importance of quality of life, the absence of well-being and the role of socio-economic and structural factors. Great weight is attributed to the experience of illness through self-reports and to socio-economic factors and definitions of need from users themselves.

The notion of need reflects people's identity, the extent to which they have access to other resources and the perceived legitimacy they have in utilising services. With regard to mental health, such subjectivity is frequently extended in a way which does not separate out the illness from the 'self'. In clinical terms,[1] conditions such as, say, 'depression', can be characterised essentially as a categorical set of mutually exclusive symptoms. These include depressed mood, and/or greatly diminished interest in, or pleasure from, normal activities and one or more of the following: significant weight loss or gain, sleep disturbance, feelings of excessive guilt or worthlessness, reduced ability to think or concentrate, or indecisiveness, retardation or agitation, fatigue or loss of energy, recurrent thoughts of death or suicidal thoughts or actions. This categorisation may bear little relationship to the experience of the person presenting with problems such as depression, which has also been conceptualised as an existential condition that involves a loss or reconfiguration of the self, and so as a distinctive illness career (Karp 1994).

What demarcates the experience of mental health problems from other chronic conditions is the impossibility of dissociating the self from the condition (Fabrega and Manning 1972). For the sufferer, the experience may be of inchoate feelings of distress and the certainty that something is very wrong. Negotiation of the illness identity that follows from this is often problematic. Many sufferers of psychological problems may actively reject the diagnostic labels to which health care professionals adhere (Rogers *et al.* 1993). Lewis (1995) offers an interpretation of sufferer's responses to the diagnosis of depression that emphasises the search for meaning, and the tension between individual and social explanations in the cause of depression. This ambiguous status of a condition, for which help is sought, is the context within which access to and contact with services is negotiated and responded to. The expression of psychosocial pain at the interface with services is problematic. Services tend towards providing options of a split between the psyche and the soma. However, for some groups in the population, the connectedness between the expression of physical and psychosocial pain cannot be parcelled out in this way.

Conclusion

Service provision illuminates a number of facets of social divisions and inequalities in mental health. At times, services have been seen as the epicentre of the unequal and marginalised status of mad people. In this regard, the large mental hospitals provided a critical focus for society's treatment of this group. The focus on services provision and utilisation has detracted attention from sources of social exclusion operating in wider society. The ways in which services influence mental health status and the expression of mental health need are neglected aspects of contemporary mental health knowledge. Whether or not services ameliorate or promote well-being has also to be judged against the balance between coercion and voluntarism during service contact. Finally, an objectified notion of 'mental illness' obscures the extent to which the supply and demand of mental health services has the potential to meet need, which is subjectively expressed by individuals.

4

Primary care, mental health and inequalities

Introduction

In the previous chapter, we argued for abandoning an understanding of inequalities that separates the impact of external social conditions on mental health from that created by service contact. We began to show the way in which these two sources of influence are linked. In daily life, service contact and the variegated experience and impact of community stressors are not parcelled out as separate domains. Experientially, they coexist for people. Moreover, whilst the point has frequently been made that services, given their cost, have a modest impact on levels of morbidity and mortality, there are a number of subtle ways in which services have the potential either to ameliorate or to perpetuate illness trajectories and social divisions. Nowhere is this more apparent than in the arena of primary health care, the point in the health care system which interfaces routinely with the public.

A second related aspect of our argument is that the interrelationship between services and mental disorders, and the consequent creation and maintenance of inequalities, is construct-specific. Primary care has been principally associated with the diagnosis and management of 'depression' and 'anxiety', the so-called 'common' or 'minor' 'mental disorders'. There have been increased calls for greater attention being paid to those with 'major mental disorders', particularly in relation to their physical needs, and for the participation of primary care in the management of these 'enduring mental health problems'. Primary care is restricted in its remit for managing these disorders by the prescribing mandates set by Consultant Psychiatrists and by practices such as the 'care management' approach, which are directed by specialist staff in hospital-based or community mental health teams.

Thus, the focus in this chapter is mainly (though not exclusively) on the management of those diagnosed with depression and/or anxiety. These have been strongly associated with issues of gender inequality and primary care has, to an extent, contributed to a particular, feminised view of 'depression'. A focus on the interface with this part of the health care system also illuminates those adverse or oppressive contexts that influence people to seek help from medicine. As a result, primary care services label and then transform personal troubles or psychosocial misery into an individual medical condition of 'depression'.

Primary care holds an important strategic position, as it remains the point in the health care system governed by an explicit commitment to equity. It is the main site where the British NHS meets its obligation to provide a service free at the point of need. Recent 'official' British health policy has attempted to give greater weight (and responsibility) to the role of primary care in the provision of care and the management of mental health problems. Within this policy context, primary care is offered as a vehicle of equalisation. It does this in two ways, first by providing, in theory at least, a means of treatment to those who seek help from a General Practitioner (GP) or other primary health care professional and, second, by providing a standard gateway for equitable access to secondary care.

Access to these first-line services is viewed as having a potential positive influence on the severity, and prevalence, of morbidity. Goldberg and Huxley's (1980) suggestion, that, over a period of a year, more than 90 per cent of patients considered to be suffering from a mental disorder made contact with their GP, has been taken as a key reference point from which to hang a policy of mental health promotion and prevention. Consequently, primary care has been targeted as the agency for the secondary prevention of mental health problems (by seeking to identify them early and nip them in the bud with optimal treatment).

The first point of contact with the health service defines psychosocial ills in a particular way. These are not only 'managed' by the patient and their doctor, they also are shaped by the socio-economic context in which that relationship is situated. For example, primary care has been a particular target for drug company marketing (Lyon 1996) (see Chapter 8) and it is where multiple social disadvantage is expressed as personal distress, which is then medicalised. As we discuss in detail below, this is achieved both through attempts by policy makers to promote 'depression' and 'anxiety' as conditions on a par with other medical diseases, and through a style of professional–'patient' interaction which reinforces a medicalised view of personal misery. Given that primary care forms an intersection between populations and individuals on the one hand and formal service provision and social conditions on the other, it is a useful site for illuminating the fact that inequalities in health status and inequalities in service provision are recursively related.

In this chapter, we draw heavily on two empirical studies undertaken at the University of Manchester (Rogers *et al.* 2001; Rogers *et al.* 2002). In the first part of the chapter, after describing briefly the changing direction of primary care in relation to mental health and inequalities, we discuss the way in which a primary care focus has contributed to the medicalisation of depression. We explore the gendered effects of iatrogenic drug prescribing and how such a policy met resistance from social forces that no longer accepted a solution that resulted in widespread addiction and the oppression of women.

We also draw upon a study looking at the negotiation of depression in primary care work. This qualitative investigation challenges the view that mental health problems 'out there' are fixed prior to contact with services and are simply responded to in a prescribed and uniform way by primary care. Instead, the study illuminates the impossibility of separating service delivery and the way in which psychosocial distress is framed. Both patients and practitioners are compelled to work within the parameters of given organisational and conceptual restraints which shape a particular response and outcome during individual consultations. This process necessarily (albeit unintentionally) reinforces an individualised and medicalised view of psychological distress, creating a distance of understanding from the personal and social contexts implicated in the genesis of mental health problems.

In the second part of the chapter we consider a wider, politically orchestrated policy initiative – the ways in which new primary care organisations (Primary Care Groups and Trusts) have attempted to implement a 'quality improvement' agenda. This is one way in which official policy makers have attempted, via a 'top down' approach, to improve the 'Cinderella' status of mental health.

The changing role of primary care

The health policy significance of primary care has expanded considerably over the last four decades. Primary care has: increased in its capacity to deliver services; been central to health policy; and included a broad network of professionals. This has been a globalising trend. For example, Eastern Europe has moved largely from a system with no GPs and dominated by specialist-led 'polyclinics', to developing a whole new system of GP-based health care. The USA health care system has moved from being entirely specialist-based, to one in which more than 50 per cent of people with a health plan are obliged to see a primary care practitioner as first contact. It has been recognised, too, in developing countries that primary care should predominate, instead of relying on building more large hospitals.

With these converging global trends in mind, we use the UK as our example for analysing inequalities in mental health because of the growth and importance attributed to the primary health care sector over a number of years and its place in a State-funded system of health care with the aspiration of providing an equitable system of health care. In the UK, traditionally, mental health has held an ambiguous status in primary care policy and delivery. Until recently, its role in mental health has been traditionally overshadowed by secondary care or 'specialist' services. This has manifested itself in relation to both knowledge and service models, which have been derived predominantly from the secondary sector rather than being created afresh in primary care.

Primary care workers and their lobbyists have had relatively little involvement in the development of the mental health agenda at a national policy level. Comments from the specialist sector about mental health (including mental health in primary care) have tended to predominate in the Department of Health and in local service configuration. This lack of political influence at the centre of health policy has meant that primary care mental health work often has been driven by the assumptions and expectations of the secondary care sector.

Thus, one important dimension of inequity has been that, until recently, a distinctive primary care focus has failed to emerge about mental health. This conclusion is seen most explicitly in relation to the example of the screening and diagnosis of mental disorders. GPs have been targeted for failing to detect appropriately high levels of depression in the community. A significant amount of space is given over in the psychiatric literature to identifying why GPs fail in this regard and to measures designed to increase detection rates (e.g., Freeling *et al.* 1985; Littlejohns *et al.* 1999). However, diagnostic criteria and assumed practitioner competency are not the only factors influencing GP decision-making. In practice, primary care professionals have to consider who is available in their local network of mental health specialists. This reflects parochial resource levels rather than simply diagnostic considerations. The clients of primary care might not always place the same value on the screening and detection of mental illness as psychiatrists do. The fact that GPs are sometimes poor diagnosticians, as judged by traditional psychiatric standards, and hold views closer to lay definitions of mental health problems, means that users' preferences coincide with a perceived narrower cultural gap relating to knowledge than is the case with specialists.

Recent policy making has sought to refocus the role of primary care in tackling mental health problems. This counterbalances the disproportionate concentration on the relationship between primary and secondary care. There has been a notable shift in official policy intentions which conceptualises the role of primary care as needing to face outwards to respond to mental health need in local communities. This has more firmly placed primary care within a public health perspective of tackling mental health. The emphasis has been on the need to impact on mental health at the level of populations as well as individuals. For example, *Our Healthier Nation* (DoH 1998b) outlined an approach which placed an onus on primary care workers and other local health agencies developing strategies that can respond to both the local sources of distress and their impact on patients and potential patients.

In theory, at least, this focus is likely to address more adequately the considerable evidence of an 'iceberg' of unmet need, particularly for conditions such as post-natal depression (Whitton *et al.* 1996[1]). However, attempts to engender a 'public health focus' in relation to mental health, through approaches such as 'Community Orientated Primary Care', have proved elusive. The primary mental health agenda continues to be marginalised by primary care professionals in their work (as well as by their reliance on the dominance of secondary care). This may be, in part, because of a sense of a lack of professional control over the socio-economic causes of mental distress and the relative absence of effective clinical (i.e., individually targeted) interventions (Gillam and Miller 1997). With benzodiazepines falling into disrepute (though not being totally abandoned), antidepressants are being used increasingly as a single blunderbuss approach to all of the nuances of 'anxiety and depression' presenting in clinical consultations. And although more evidence is emerging of effective psychological interventions, these are labour intensive and unevenly available in the NHS.

Another change in the UK, which has involved substantial and rapid organisational development at the turn of the century, places primary care in an altogether more powerful strategic and structural position to instigate and carry through policy aspirations. The sector is no longer an aggregate network of individual General Practices and surgeries or health centres, but is governed by the new organisational arrangements of Primary Care Groups and Trusts (PCG/Ts). This has shifted the governance of primary care from individual practices to a local collective organisation with a superordinate managerial power-base.

PCG/Ts have also been required to implement clinical governance – the 1997 Labour Government's quality assurance measure, which displaced the internal market in the NHS. The Labour administration also set standards for different patient groups by issuing National Service Frameworks – the first one issued being about mental health, which contained a number of relevant measures relating to primary care and inequalities. We turn to an in-depth exploration of this later on in this chapter. Before that, we address our first topic – the management of 'depression'.

Managing depression in primary care

In Chapter 2, we discussed the issue of access to mental health services with reference to the inverse care law. This was mainly concerned with a population and service level analysis. We now want to turn to a 'micro' level exploration. In so doing, we draw on a qualitative study of the management of depression in primary care that one of us (AR) has undertaken, with colleagues Linda Gask, Carl May and Dianne Oliver, at the University of Manchester.

This work originated in research which explored the ways in which doctors and patients conceptualise and respond to depression as a problem in the specific organisational context of primary care. This was done by drawing on the narratives of twenty-seven patients and ten GPs recruited from ten different practices in the Greater Manchester area. Patient accounts from the semi-structured interviews illuminated the background to, and ways in which, people made contact with and experienced help-seeking, consultation and management. At the beginning of the patient interviews, respondents were asked about the experience of depression and its causes. Later, the interviews moved on to explore their use of primary care.

It is striking that whilst the need for help was pressing and anxiously sought, the overall contact with primary care was found to be of relatively little significance when set against the magnitude of experienced problems (these formed the landmarks of patients' accounts). This, in itself, signifies the inadequacy of the dominant societal response to psychosocial distress caused by social and personal injury. Clinical interventions from primary care were regarded as a benign, but relatively inconsequential, intrusion into social worlds characterised by loss and hopelessness. Subjects' lives were dominated by material and cultural disadvantage and abusive relationships, and these were sources of a deeply embedded sense of existential despair. Our respondents were, for the most part, people with multiple problems, which were largely related to occupational insecurity, poverty and social exclusion and the impact that these had on intimate relationships and on childcare. Respondents accounted for the onset of their depression in terms of being unable, in some fundamental way, to 'cope' with their everyday circumstances in the face of this pressure. One respondent observed, for example

> I became quite a recluse, I wouldn't go out of the house – working seven days a week became too much for any one person to do. I couldn't cope with work and home and everything. I was crying all the time – panic attacks.

Another point underlining the small, explicit impact of primary care contact is that sufferers spent very little time in face-to-face consultations with their doctors or other primary care professionals. Nonetheless, contact with primary care had an *implicit* significance in shaping their experiences of depression and the parameters of their expectations of help from the wider apparatus of health care.

Previous studies in different cultural and organisational contexts have pointed to relatively long periods of problem formulation and delays in seeking help for depression (Kadushin 1969; Monroe *et al.* 1991). Consistent with this previous work, respondents in this study made contact with primary care in a variety of ways and at different points in the trajectory of their depression 'careers'. Like respondents in Karp's (1994) account of depressed North Americans, those interviewed for this study constructed their experiences of being unable to cope in relation to a range of inchoate feelings.

The respondents struggled to articulate the nature of their problem and its associated distress. When conduct was seen to be out of control, it was no longer recognisable as part of the person's normal sense of self. This led to a significant degree of confusion in their formulation of the need to seek help. In a (British) culture that prizes a degree of reticence in the expression of emotional states, to behave in an explosive or chaotic way itself leads to further anxiety. This confusion and lack of control is expressed here by one of the respondents:

> I just went out of control... I just knocked everything off the side in the kitchen and things got smashed all over the floor. And this was just not me, you know? I'm not that type of person, and afterwards I thought... I was picking this stuff up, and I thought 'why have I done this?' You know, 'what has possessed me to do this?' I think it was just sheer frustration, knowing there was something wrong but I didn't know what to do about it. So, I don't know, it just all seemed to get on top of me.

Anticipating and negotiating contact with GPs

An assessment of what can be expected from health services by patients is based on prior contact. Under ordinary circumstances of physical illness, patients learn to fit in with what is required of them from prior experience of what health professionals consider to be a legitimate illness. In particular, people learn to differentiate and modify their presentation of feelings to an adjudged degree, otherwise they risk not being treated or not being confirmed in the sick role (Telles and Pollack 1981).

This implies the existence of a mutuality and predictability in the relationship between patients and service providers which is anticipated consciously or unconsciously by both parties (Rogers *et al.* 1999). However, in relationship to people diagnosed with depression needing to access primary care, this assumption cannot be taken for granted since the problems in question are not unambigiously medical in nature. Respondents reported that they experienced anxiety in waiting to see the doctor and in deciding how to introduce the idea that they had a problem that they were unable to formulate clearly in their own minds. In addition, they experienced a number of other difficulties related to the 'less deserving' status assumed to apply to mental health compared to physical health problems. Some respondents, for example, felt (or anticipated) a degree of shame at presenting with what they perceived must be a psychological problem, while others felt that their problem was not really a medical problem at all.

Respondents also indicated a sense that however they construed their problem and presented it to the doctor, there was a possibility of negative and unwanted consequences of the consultation. In relation to these contingencies, a reluctance to disclose a fragile sense of being able to cope was identifiable. One man made his own gendered link in this sort of dilemma when he told the interviewer that his reason for delaying contact with the GP was because 'it's not easy to admit you can't cope, you know, when you are a grown mature man'.

The decision to consult the doctor did not necessarily imply a fully medicalised view of personal troubles. In fact, for many of our respondents, GPs were consulted because the latter constituted the *only* source of help that seemed accessible at a particular moment. However people with distress see their problems, they may have only a Hobson's Choice about their amelioration:

> It was a general feeling of decline and to the point where I did go and see him [the GP] I was emotionally right at rock bottom, you know? I needed to go and speak to him, to somebody and see if something could be done.

The decision to consult the GP was also formed around the perceived appropriateness of people's troubles to fit the set of norms and values about help-seeking and treatment expected in primary care. There was a degree of pessimism about the extent to which the ministrations of primary care physicians would actually be able to help and there were reported pressures for social and personal problems to be viewed in individualised terms.

I just think, what is the point of going back to see him? He can't do anything. Nobody can do anything, even the tablets it's just something I've got to work through myself.

In this context of respondents feeling that primary care could not do much to alleviate a problem, they also intimated an internalised lack of legitimacy about consulting. In this regard, people felt that they had the 'wrong' type of problem and that the 'right' sort of problem was essentially a physical one:

When I get there, I get the feeling that there's nothing wrong with me. I wish I had got something physical to show. Sometimes, when we are in the car, I hope we crash. I really have hoped we crash and that I wouldn't die, but that something would happen that would give me a *real*reason for being off work and feeling the way I do.

Primary care held out a threat, as well as a source of support. This was related to the threat of coercion we discussed in Chapter 2. People undergoing feelings of distress and a loss of control and personal normality worry at times that psychiatric compulsion may lie just ahead. They also may feel that service contact may amplify, not diminish, their loss of control. This might disrupt an already fragile sense of self. For example, one female respondent stated that she avoided contact with her GP because, 'I'm frightened of going on to something stronger, I don't want to become addicted or anything. That's why I'm really frightened of drugs.'

Establishing the nature of the problem for which help was being sought was also an intrinsic problem in these accounts of trajectories of help-seeking. The circumstances in which the label of 'depression' was attributed to people presenting such problems to the general practitioner constituted a point of passage in which the person became, to a greater or lesser extent, a patient. This constituted a shift in their self-identity. For some, the act of diagnosis by the GP had little significance. Indeed, it confirmed a view that was already well established in the sufferer. For other respondents, entering the clinical domain had a greater impact in terms of shaping the ontological status of having depression.

Some had no prior recognition that their problem was one of depression and the attribution of this diagnostic label involved reconceptualising ideas about illness and adapting to them. For example, one of our respondents attended her GP for a seemingly different problem:

> It sort of came out in the topic of conversation over something else. I thought I had shingles on my back, and as we were talking it just came out and it's just developed from there. And when she [the doctor] suggested something I thought, 'well, yeah, maybe this might help'. And, I was quite accepting of it and relieved that hopefully something might be able to help me.

The medicalisation of misery in routine primary care work

The impact of contact with primary care in shaping and responding to existential and social problems that become constituted as a medical condition, called 'depression', is illuminated further when we look at how clinicians constructed accounts of patient presentations. The reshaping of the subjective experience of the (patient's) self is missing in medical accounts. Whilst misery is highly personal and individuated for the sufferer, in the experience of clinicians the understanding and treatment of 'depression' is simply a routinised part of 'doing' everyday family medicine.

For doctors, the management of depression is, unsurprisingly perhaps, first and foremost part of medical work. For them, the central issue was recognising and dealing with the *pathology* that the patient presented. Historically, GPs have emphasised that theirs is a clinical discipline that relies on understanding and 'knowing' the patient (May and Mead 1999). The consultation is the cornerstone upon which this rests, and in which the patient comes to be understood, not only in reductionist or objectifying terms about pathology (though it includes these) but also as a person located in a psychosocial context who also demands to be understood. So, in relation to a patient quoted above, their GP asserted:

> GP: She has a relationship breakdown because her husband ... I think he's a first cousin [it's an] arranged marriage. He was very good with her at the start, [when] he came to this country. She had a son, and after that he started to be more interested in settling in this country and in looking after his parents back home than taking the responsibility of [name] and her child. And, you know, that is the basic problem. Obviously she became irritable and depressed. She has reactive depression and I'm hoping the situation will resolve ... she has some symptoms of anxiety and depression. She was irritable, was crying and losing concentration, and

having problems looking after the baby, not sleeping, a lot of tension headaches and aches and pains in her body.

Interviewer: What's your role in managing the problem?

GP: I asked her to see the counsellor but I don't think that she has been to see her, and I started her on antidepressants.

The extent to which the experience of depression was formed around social and personal difficulties, in social contexts where sufferers were faced with multiple sources of disadvantage, were well understood by clinicians. In the circumstances that many sufferers found themselves, depression and depressive symptoms were construed as 'natural' responses to the problems that they faced. Doctors recognised that the sources of the symptoms they encountered were often external to the sufferer[2] – the sufferer had approached them seeking clinical help for a personal problem.

Nonetheless, however much the profession of general practice has focused on ideas about 'holistic' care, and however much individual clinicians in this study recognised the idiosyncratic circumstances that led to the patient's presentation, the pathology of depression lay at the centre of their activities. This attributed tension between the pathology and the individuated experience of depression, and their amplification by, and intelligibility within, the social context in which sufferers were located, runs through the doctors' accounts. They appreciated the impact of these wider social and psychological factors on the experiences of sufferers. But in a short primary care consultation, it is the clinical synopsis, the abbreviated account of symptoms, *the diagnosis*, which drive practice. In this medical process, ontology and subjectivity are certainly considered but they are then pushed to the margins of medical consideration.

The form and direction of the medical narratives collected reveal patterns of clinical reasoning. In the case of our clinician respondents, however much they constituted depression as a product of the social and psychological experiences of sufferers, they emphasised depression as a medical problem and depicted miserable people as patients like any other. Pilgrim *et al.* (1997) suggests that a categorical diagnostic emphasis in mental health referrals is central to the ease and control GPs feel they have in securing a desired referral outcome. In this context, clinicians asserted that if the structural constraints they experienced were less pressing, then they might respond to depression in a different way. Here, a GP comments:

> Persaud [a populist psychiatrist in the mass media] was saying 'wouldn't it be interesting if the GP could spend an hour instead of the therapist, who would the patient prefer to spend the hour with?' I thought that was an interesting thought, not that I've got an hour!

So, to respond to the sufferer in a way that extended beyond the prescription of routine antidepressants and attempted to engage deeply with the patient's problem was not possible for the GP.

Differing sources of patient and doctor pessimism

Clinicians' accounts were underpinned by a pessimism that ran in parallel to that evinced in patients' stories. Where patients were pessimistic about the prospects of being helped by doctors, GPs were themselves pessimistic about their capacity to help the patient within their own practice or by referral to secondary services. While much of the primary care literature stresses the gatekeeping function of general practice, this was a real problem for these doctors. They recognised that there was little that they could do for patients beyond providing antidepressant drugs. Secondary care services were overwhelmed by the 'seriously mentally ill' – routinely depressed people had little power to compete with them. Also, as psychiatry is mainly driven by drug treatments (see Chapters 8 and 9), Consultant Psychiatrists only have access to the same solutions on their prescription pads as GPs and psychological treatments are sparsely available:

> Interviewer: What's the waiting list to see a psychologist?
>
> GP: It's about four months at the moment. So that's a problem. A lot of people end up being put on medication. Perhaps if they could see a psychologist within two weeks then they wouldn't need medication. But there is a feeling that you've got to do something – counselling. That's only recently started, so I'm not sure how that's going to work out. So it's something we need to evaluate to see how useful it is for people with depression. And then there's psychiatry, but that's not particularly useful for people with depression unless they're seriously ill because the waiting list is so long. Psychiatric services are just swamped with people with major mental illness.

GPs were at pains to point to the unevenness of secondary care services, and the potential unreliability of those which existed. Access to care was a crucial problem. While GPs were concerned about their poor access to specialist services, it was not always clear what they hoped that these would achieve. They recognised the importance of time, and in some accounts there was a suggestion that in depression there was a trajectory of recovery that was revealed by time itself. A minority of GPs focused on the extent to which psychogenic disease itself had a 'natural history' that in individual instances could be routinely engaged through conventional treatments. The principal feature of GP accounts of depression was, in fact, how little they had to say about it. Depression is one of the staples of GP practice, routinely treated with drugs, and sometimes through referral to counsellors. For the most part, our clinician respondents itemised their activities with specific patients in terms of their 'clinical' history and trajectory through the structures of primary care, while clearly personally distancing themselves from the kinds of experience that patients presented. Instead, their complaints were about the poor services that they had to assist them in dealing with populations which were subject to a massive range of multiple disadvantages, when it was difficult to distinguish between despair and depression.

With regard to ongoing management, in both the patients' and GPs' accounts of depression, arrangements for continuing contact tended to conform to the routines established for other common conditions in primary care. There was little evidence of special arrangements to ensure ongoing care, and re-attendance in primary care was for repeat prescribing or sick notes picked up from the receptionist. There was little to suggest from patients' accounts that they made arrangements with their GPs for continuing contact during or after, for example, any period of counselling.

In summary, expectations about primary care from both patients and clinicians in our study could be described as 'low but realistic'. As with other conditions, mental health need often translates into whether a problem can be managed with available technology, treatment and resources. This is evident at a systemic level within primary care. It has been suggested that the lower level of psychosomatic complaints in British compared to French primary care may be a function of a capitation fee system (where a yearly lump sum is paid for each patient) which inhibits the expression of such illness compared with the illness norms which are able to be expressed under a fee-for-service system (Williams 1983).

In our study, case management resources were generally limited within primary care to the prescribing of antidepressants and an assessment of what was wrong. There were few, if any, expectations that primary care could tackle the root causes of the problem, which were seen to lie outside a traditional medical model of illness. Whilst care in general practice has often been portrayed as an active process of negotiation between lay and professional knowledge, this takes place against the less obvious routines and assumptions about the way in which primary care is organised and limited (by financial resources and clinical effectiveness). The acceptance of this by both patients and professionals coalesced into a consensus around sparse attendance and familiar short routines when using primary care.

Furthermore, this study illuminates the poverty of viewing access in relation to just practice position and organisation (location, appointment systems, waiting times, choice of physician). The problems people had in accessing care related to process rather than structure. They included difficulties in formulating and expressing a mental health problem in an organisational context where the presentation of physical illness, and its management, is the assumed norm. The threat of a further loss of control, anticipated in the possible response of the GP, inhibited or delayed contact being made.

Prescribed psychotropic drugs and the medicalisation of misery

The main form of treatment, psychotropic drugs, tends to be viewed negatively by patients but the latter may also accept the role of pills fatalistically. In our study, patients were seemingly passive recipients of the clinician's treatment decisions and the main activity that this involved was medication. Some patients were reluctant to accept medication, and eight reported discontinuing it, either because of side-effects or because it failed to deal with their perceived problems. Similarly, other research into patients' perceptions of taking pills or tablets suggests that medication is viewed not as alleviating some sort of pathology but performing another function. Medication is viewed as a 'prop' or 'lifeline' – something to keep going in the face of chronic difficulties, or as a 'standby' – to keep in reserve to get through a short-term crisis.

Taking psychotropic drugs is seen by recipients as having social risks which cross the boundary between warrantable behaviour (treatment for illness) and moral culpability (not coping and being reliant on the 'crutch of a drug') (Gabe and Lipschitz-Phillips 1984). Consequently, some patients who have crossed this boundary may be more ready to accept what is on offer from primary care simply because they no longer feel they have a mandate to challenge this. Thus, there seems to be a degree of acceptance that medication is the main or only treatment available within primary care. Additionally, and notwithstanding the popularity of talking treatments in primary care, which arguably have more connectedness to the everyday realities of peoples' lives, medication continues to play a central role in perpetuating inequalities in treatment, particularly in primary care.

When compared with other psychotropic medication, such as major tranquillisers, antidepressants receive more positive evaluations, perhaps because they are often prescribed by GPs in voluntary community settings (Rogers *et al.* 1993). Nonetheless, there is a widespread public perception that antidepressants are addictive and should not be given to depressed people. Many patients treated with antidepressants in primary care stop taking them prematurely (Priest *et al.* 1996).

It is clear that the 'acceptance' of antidepressants is, to a large degree, a poor substitute for dealing more directly with the social and personal troubles that arise out of familial, social and economic conditions. The widespread use of the newer antidepressants, such as Prozac, can be seen as a reinforcement of the medicalisation of psychosocial problems, in the wake of a legitimation crisis over the widespread use of benzodiazepine minor tranquillisers. In the latter instance, the iatrogenic risks were seen as too high to sustain, and the levels and effects of addiction on women, in particular, came to be seen as socially unacceptable (Gabe and Bury 1996; Gabe and Bury 1991).

In one sense, the prescription of minor tranquillisers by GPs could have been viewed as a form of 'under-medicalisation', as it was a response to vague symptoms ('tired all the time'), rather than to distinct conditions or 'proper' mental illnesses. Consequently, the *ad hoc* and widespread nature of prescribing (a key focus of criticism) became associated with a lack of specialist and appropriate technical competence on the part of GPs. By contrast, the emergence of a new generation of antidepressants has been more specifically linked to the diagnosis of depression within primary care, even though in practice it is prescribed for a range of different conditions. Indeed, currently the newer antidepressants appear to have simply replaced benzodiazepines as a general nostrum for distress. Depending on their dose level, they claim to lift mood or to have an anxiolytic effect. Popular texts have emphasised the biological connection with improvements in feelings of self-worth and, in general terms, the drugs were promoted as offering a more empowering imagery than the 'housewife hooked' on minor tranquillisers. Drugs like Prozac were advertised as having positive and normalising attributes, not only lifting depressed mood and demoralisation in the sick but making the well feel even better (Lyons 1996).

Medicalisation as a site of resistance: gender and race considered

Examples given above point to the way in which medicalisation is a means of promoting inequalities. Through individual diagnosis and treatment, it pacifies at the individual level and disconnects personal problems from the social contexts in which they arise. Feminist analyses have, in the same vein, revealed the gendered nature of constructs of official and medical notions of madness (Chesler 1972). The constructions of those suffering from 'depression' or 'anxiety' promote and feed into wider cultural notions about those in receipt of the diagnoses. The transmission of these ideas as common currency in popular and medical knowledge is aptly shown by the analysis of media coverage about women taking minor tranquillisers (Gabe *et al.* 1991).

Medicalisation is also a site of resistance for the marginalised at a collective and individual level. Strategies of empowerment in response to the oppressive situation of women in modern society have been central to the analyses provided by feminist-inspired social scientists (Orbach 1978, 1986; Showalter 1987; Ussher 1991). These analyses have impacted upon or reflected other social processes (e.g., media representations of women's roles and aspirations) within civil society. This vociferous and notable resistance, in being associated predominantly with women, has perhaps overshadowed other ways in which social injury arising from iatrogenesis and medicalisation is managed. This is reflected in the seemingly low rates of use of primary care services by Afro-Caribbean groups and of their diagnosed depression.

The reasons for apparently relatively low rates of consultation for depression amongst Afro-Caribbean groups, and black women in particular, are likely to be multi-causal. They implicate the labelling practices of professionals and pathways into care (e.g., police referrals), which reflect the wider (white) public perception of mental disorder amongst black people. However, the coping strategies of individuals may link quite specifically to ethnic identity and social roles. Studies exploring the way in which black women manage mental distress and interact with primary care illuminate the role of their identity and social position when negotiating treatment and management of mental health problems in primary care.

The availability and involvement in paid work, the nature of social support and function of religious beliefs have been cited as elements explaining differential patterns of the use of tranquillisers prescribed in primary care. In the early 1980s, Gabe and Thorogood (1986) found that 'indigenous' white working-class women were more likely to use benzodiazepines in the long term compared to a group of West Indian-born women. Black women were more likely to have supportive older children living at home and a full-time job. The latter, it has been suggested, may arise from employment being seen in the eyes of black women as enabling. Black women may hold a greater value on this than their white counterparts and place an emphasis on financial independence and work as a social support mechanism and effective coping strategy when dealing with personal adversity.

A more recent qualitative study of depression amongst Afro-Caribbean women (Edge 2002) has found that lower rates of formally diagnosed depression may be accounted for by strong social imperatives to normalise distress when faced with difficult times in life. A resistance to psychiatric labelling, aspirations for their children, and religious affiliation emerge as powerful counters to entering the sick role and receiving and accepting a diagnosis of depression amongst the Afro-Caribbean women interviewed in the study. In line with the discussion on recursivity above, this study also suggests that access to services such as psychological counselling and other resources, which might assist with dealing with social injury, may, to an extent, be countered by such normalising strategies towards depression. GPs and other health professionals may act to reinforce self-reliance and inhibit requests for assistances and services from other sources by failing to identify and label distress as depression requiring treatment. Whether this 'under-diagnosis' and 'failure to treat' is good or bad is, of course, a moot point, but what is clear is that the cultural norms and aspirations of being a black woman in a white society impacts on primary service utilisation when distress is experienced.

Clinical governance in primary care

We now turn away from inequalities and reactions to them, which are located at the interface with General Practice and primary care mental health professionals, to exploring the way in which mental health fares in relation to other conditions when it comes to delivering optimal service provision. The *National Service Framework For Mental Health* (NSF) published by the government in 1999 presents primary care organisation with a quasi-statutory obligation to implement particular standards in mental health care. Through the Mental Health NSF, which was informed by a multi-stakeholder 'reference group', the Labour Government introduced an expanded focus on mental health inequalities and the promotion of mental health (Tyrer 1999). The Mental Health NSF for the first time established a set of officially sanctioned minimum standards, to which those in the health and social welfare community, through 'performance management', are expected to conform (DoH 1999).

The government envisaged that the implementation of the NSF, and the service development it required, would underpin the operation of proposed mental health legislation to replace the 1983 Mental Health Act. Like other clinical areas included under the umbrella of clinical governance, the NSF for mental health is informed by the ethos of evidence-based practice. The seven standards issued under the rubric of the Mental Health NSF cover the spectrum of the promotion of mental health and management of mental illness across community, secondary and primary care settings.[3]

The seven standards cover five aspects: mental health promotion; primary care; access to services; effective care for those diagnosed as having a severe mental illness; and suicide prevention. The key aim for primary care is to: 'deliver better primary mental health care and to ensure consistent advice and help for people with mental health needs, including primary care services for individuals with severe mental illness'. This position subsequently was reinforced and elaborated in further prescriptive guidance (the *Mental Health Policy Implementation Guide*, DoH 2001).

Under the NSF, primary care has the responsibility to ensure that any service user who contacts their primary health care team with a common mental health problem should have their mental health needs identified and assessed. Primary care is also charged with ensuring that such patients are offered effective treatments, including referral to specialist services if required. According to Gask *et al.* (2000) these require primary care groups and trusts to lead on the following aspects: organising training for primary care staff; developing PCG-wide clinical guidelines on prescribing protocols; and providing information to practices about available resources (social welfare and voluntary resources).

Rival conditions? Coronary heart disease and mental health

We now turn to the study, carried out at the National Primary Care Research and Development Centre at the University of Manchester, in which views of key respondents within PCG/Ts, charged with implementing the policy assumptions, were explored. This study focused on the standing attributed by the respondents to the mental health NSF standards, in the policy context of clinical governance. In particular, we examined how mental health was dealt with in comparison to Coronary Heart Disease (CHD), which was also the subject of a National Service Framework introduced shortly after the launch of the Mental Health NSF.

The government justification for prioritising mental health and CHD, as the first two Service Frameworks to be introduced by the Department of Health, was that they were considered to 'cover two of the most significant causes of ill-health and disability in England'. However, in terms of levels of activities and plans for the future, it was found that the mental health agenda did not hold the same status as that of Coronary Heart Disease within PCGs. The latter were much more likely to have identified CHD rather than mental health as a priority topic for improving clinical care (by a ratio of nearly 3:1). Moreover, whilst many PCG/Ts had identified mental health as a topic requiring improvement, when it came to implementing *actual plans* for improvement, mental health lagged behind CHD.

Box 4.1 illustrates the differences in implementation of the Coronary Heart Disease NSF compared with that of mental health.

Box 4.1   Coronary heart disease and mental health

	CHD	MH
Most practices have met some criteria already	yes	no
Most practices familiar with some of the NSF content	yes	no
Protocol and guideline driven	yes	no
Seen as mostly primary rather than secondary care led	yes	no
Seen as easily measurable/something to count	yes	no
Requires more partnership working and networking	no	yes
Greater potential for primary care to be proactive	yes	no
Some skills/staff necessary available in primary care	yes	no
Necessary infrastructure (registers, etc.) available	yes	no
Focus on systems of care rather than individual practices	no	yes
Greater potential focus for quality assurance	yes	no
Allow PCG/Ts to assess progress against baselines	yes	yes
Enable best practice to be rolled-out	yes	yes
Potential role for clinical governance facilitators	yes	yes

The question this information begs is *why* mental health was comparatively more problematic as a clinical governance issue than that created by the CHD NSF. The narratives offered by respondents suggested that the latter clearly had an advantage over mental health, in that it was seen as a biomedical, clinical issue *par excellence*, which, with only modest efforts, GPs could embrace. By contrast, mental health suffered from being something that was much more uncertain. Its biopsychosocial complexity is challenging to medical practitioners, and PCG/Ts are expected to instigate strategic change in broadly defined areas around multi-agency working. This point is brought out here by a respondent in the study:

> The CHD NSF . . . we feel there's a definite bit in that, that's quite didactic and tells you what standards primary care should be achieving. The Mental Health NSF was much less sort of immediately directive. I mean, you know most of us GPs can cope with being told you know, 'You've got to get this blood level or that, or use this drug or that thing and monitor this and measure that' and that's pretty easy, you can put a handle on that and check whether you've done it. The mental health one wasn't quite so obvious, so I suspect, yes, most feel much more engaged by the CHD one, than by the mental health one. (PCG Clinical governance lead).

The essence of the high status attributable to the NSFs, within a broader clinical governance agenda, was the demand for definitive and measurable outcomes. As one respondent said, 'I would put 'them (NSFs) in the first division of priorities mainly because the standards they contain are so quantifiable and measurable'. In this regard, the less tangible mental health NSF was seen as posing a much greater challenge than the CHD framework. One PCG mental health lead referred to the mental health standards as 'mum and apple pie' and another that their main aim was to raise the profile of mental health in primary care, rather than to *actually achieve* specified outcomes. One respondent compared the likely practice implications of measurability as follows:

> I mean, going back to coronary heart disease, the practices know that they will be sharing this CHD data at a later date because there is something we can count... I keep looking at mental health NSF and say, 'how will we design some sort of project around this, which is going to have measurable outcomes?', each time I look at it I can't come up with the answer. (PCG clinical governance lead).

The problem of producing credible performance outcomes was linked, in respondents' accounts, to a scepticism about the evidence-base upon which the mental NSF was predicated. Again negative comparisons were made with CHD 'with CHD it's all around the evidence'. A transmitted lack of enthusiasm for engagement with the mental health agenda was also related to the problems mental health seemed to pose for GPs as part of their everyday practice. The disadvantage that this created for mental health is expressed here by the mental health lead of one PCT:

> I think its true to say that many GPs are less knowledgeable about mental health than many specialities. The problem with the actual treatments for things like anxiety and neuroses is that they are chronic conditions, which take up huge amounts of time and therefore that brings pressure, because you don't have a huge amount of time. So it's a kind of a 'heart sink' subject in itself. It's not as if it's not something where you wake up in the morning thinking 'oh I've got six people with mental health problems on my surgery list today whoopee!'... people quite often want it to go away and for someone else to take over because it's difficult, it's emotional. Therefore trying to actually face the problem, seeing how big the problem is... is quite overwhelming. (PCT mental health lead)

These perceived weaknesses interfered with the PCG/Ts' imperative to show rapid improvements in health services, which reinforced
the bias away from mental health becoming a clinical governance
priority:

> We've got two competing agendas. There's the mental health bit
> and there's the ischaemic heart bit. Both say 'o yeah they're top
> priority'...And there's the danger they're [GPs] going to get over-
> whelmed...they can't see the wood for the trees and they say 'forget
> it'...So that's why we've very much gone for the ischaemic heart
> disease...We want them to see the benefit in terms of patient care that
> they're providing. (PCG Chief office)

We can see from the above quotations that although the National
Service Framework for Mental Health marked a new phase in
mental health policy making, providing, for the first time, a quality
standards template designed to ensure appropriate and high standards of service delivery, CHD standards lend themselves more
readily to quantification. This makes the CHD NSF more acceptable
to clinicians and relatively easy to introduce as a clinical governance
topic, which might generate rapid results. In contrast, the study findings raised questions about the appropriateness of indicators and
standard-based approaches for mental health problems, which remain
only precariously medicalised. In relation to mental health, 'the tail
wags the dog', in so far as indicators and standards are attempting
to drive a relatively ill-developed agenda about mental health in
primary care.

In confronting the National Service Framework for Mental
Health, those responsible for clinical governance in PCG/Ts were
forced to engage with the pragmatic difficulties which arise from an
underlying tension. The status of knowledge underpinning mental
health service provision and the complex nature of mental health
care itself had to be addressed. As we point out throughout this
book, both of these are controversial and, thus, particularly taxing
for GPs and primary care managers who only deal with mental
health as one part of their lives and, when they do, it is often experienced as a woolly, perplexing or even demoralising topic.

Recent work (Dixon 2000) has highlighted the problems faced by
GPs in resolving the gap between the medical model of mental illness,
taught in medical schools and reinforced by the pharmaceutical
lobby, and the reality of mental health problems they see in practice.

(The extent of influence of the drug companies as a dominant source of information for doctors is discussed in Chapter 8.) What constitutes an appropriate outcome in mental health practice is highly contested, compared to general medicine. For example, it is ambiguous whether 'observable' outcomes, based on standardised interviews and 'objective' measurement, are more appropriate outcomes than those based on subjective patient experience (Henderson *et al.* 1999). Moreover, there is a growing acceptance of the need for eclectic or plural 'menu' approaches to mental health. These different approaches construct the nature of mental health problems in different ways. This creates a tension between a managerial or bureaucratic need for specified evidence-based practice, which has readily measured outcomes, and the operational obligation to respond to a diffuse set of, sometimes indeterminate, personal and social needs, which are framed in different ways by different professional approaches to mental health work.[4] The aspiration to harness a variety of health and social care resources, which respond to the diverse needs of individuals, is given official endorsement in the Mental Health NSF Standards. (Standard 1 about mental health promotion and Standard 6 about carers are particularly relevant in this regard.) Thus, it is not only that mental health work is pluralistic and complex, constructing need and outcomes in various ways. It is also the case that the NSF itself encourages a broad psychosocial perspective of some of its standards.

The inclusion of a broader population focus in mental health care, in the NSF, expands enormously a traditional clinical frame of reference. For example, GPs usually think of the aggregate needs and demands of individual patients on 'their list'. By contrast, the NSF is asking PCG/Ts to see a whole local community as their remit and to think not just about common and severe mental disorders 'on GPs' lists', but aspects of social policy (such as social exclusion). As we suggested earlier, this creates a pragmatic conundrum for those charged with implementing mental health standards in the normative context of evidenced-based practice in other clinical areas (such as CHD).

This study, then, illustrates the subtle organisational processes that indirectly marginalise mental health problems compared with other conditions dealt with by the health and welfare system, despite conscious attempts to reverse the inequitable status of mental health by official policy makers.

Conclusion

At a micro-level, the practices of primary care professionals and their interactions with individuals who consult with despair and distress are, as we have seen, shaped by both the immediate resources and context within which primary care professionals and patients operate, as well as wider influences. The latter include macro socio-economic influences such as drug company profit and oppressive forces of poverty, patriarchy and racism.

The ambivalence of people consulting with mental health problems, the tenuous legitimation of a medicalised response to the oppression associated with gender and race at a collective and individual level all point to the salience of primary care as a barometer of inequality and mental health. They also illuminate any attempts at its amelioration. For example, at the beginning of this chapter we pointed to the fact that despite official recognition of the need for a greater public health focus, such an approach has been difficult to establish in the context of the absence of effective interventions and an inertia governing the marginalisation of mental health in the culture of primary care work. The result is one in which currently there is little room for manoeuvre for primary care professionals beyond reinforcing a medicalised and individualised response to social injury.

In the past, the norms, values and interests of the specialist sector have largely determined primary care activity. With a shift in policy-making, which gives greater powers to providing and managing health and welfare services, this position may change. The two studies we have discussed in some depth suggest that whilst primary care seemingly is in an advantageous position to promote greater equity at the interface between the public and services, a number of subtle processes militate against this. Within a medical culture of primary care, mental health does not have the same salience, or attractiveness, as more coherent clinical entities such as Coronary Heart Disease. At the level of the doctor–patient consultation, too, there are organisational imperatives which reinforce an individualistic and medicalised response to depression. The latter, which is the commonest psychiatric diagnosis (or 'common cold' of psychiatry), both doctor and patient agree, emanates from personal and social conditions that are inadequately dealt with by a technical, medicalised response. However, both parties find it easier to perpetuate rather than challenge this response.

5

Influences on mental health inequalities across the life-span

Introduction

This chapter will address the interplay between mental health problems and social divisions during the life span. Later in the chapter, we will look at the evidence about unequal life opportunities and particular psychosocial challenges which impact on mental health in three periods during the life course (childhood, working age and old age).

To begin with, we examine some conceptual and analytical points about the life course. We then focus on the professionally contested arena of early life. Here, there is a paradox. Whilst there is a strong professional consensus that early life predicts the degree of later vulnerability to distress and dysfunction, the reasons for this prediction are disputed by professionals from different theoretical stables. Another ambiguity adds to this contestation – the direction of causality. Are socially disadvantaged people at greater risk of receiving a psychiatric diagnosis because adversity causes mental health problems? Alternatively, do the latter create social disadvantage? Could this be a circular interaction with both views of causation being true? We return to these questions recurrently below.

Inequalities and the life course

Recent research in the field of physical health and inequalities has begun to emphasise the importance of biography-in-time (Graham

2001). Time is relevant in two senses. First, inequalities may be associated (as both causes and consequences) with cumulative temporal effects. Second, a temporal frame is needed to understand delayed effects of social or environmental conditions on health.

The emphasis on biography in research about policy interventions in unequal life prospects about physical health can be contrasted with the status in mental health research of personal accounts. In mental health research, there is a particular reason why biography is important. As we noted recurrently in this book, mental health or illness always implicate the self. However, this central point has only been emphasised in some therapeutic aspects of the mental health literature (for example, psychoanalysis is a form of biographical psychology). By contrast social psychiatry has tended to omit the biographical from a biopsychosocial model – it has become in the main a bio-social discipline. As a consequence, biography has been largely absent from research on mental health and inequalities in psychiatry.

Our own research, in which accounts were taken from family members about the meaning of mental health (Rogers and Pilgrim 1997), showed that the latter is maintained or aggravated by different psychosocial processes at different points in the life-span.

Mental health problems in early life

Because we have summarised most of the relevant literature about childhood victimisation in Chapter 6, a shorter section is offered here, raising broader questions about how early life is conceptualised within professional knowledge. For biologically oriented psychiatry, pre-natal determinants (genetic inheritance and *in utero* events) have a particular salience. In its extreme form, this line of reasoning suggests that later inequalities in mental health status are preset from birth or 'wired in' to our psychological functioning. For some psychoanalytical writers (such as those influenced by the work of Klein), individual differences in inherited drives, particularly aggression, are given a central causal role. Thus, the genetic emphasis is not limited to biological psychiatry but extends to the other bodies of knowledge such as psychotherapy. For some environmentalists, the interpersonal field in very early life is germane to our understanding of later mental health. This line of reasoning can be found in the writings of some psychoanalysts (such as Winnicott and Bowlby) as well as in behaviourist psychology (such as the work of Skinner and a range of other learning theorists).

Below, we return to the question of the childhood–adulthood mental health link. Here, we briefly note some points about emotional and behavioural difficulties in childhood. Using broad-band measures of psychiatric disorder, community surveys suggest high levels of distress and dysfunction during childhood of between 11 per cent and 26 per cent, although severe problems leading to clinical presentation, or demands for specialist services, constitute around 3–6 per cent of people under 16 years of age (Bird *et al*. 1988; Costello *et al*. 1988). The higher levels in community samples suggest that childhood is an intrinsically emotionally vulnerable period, but some commentators have noted an increase in childhood problems in recent years. This might suggest that contemporary societies are creating a recurrent backdrop of increased stress upon children compared to the past.

Emotionally disturbed children tend to accrue a secondary disadvantage of poor school performance, exclusion or avoidance. This leads to lowered levels of academic achievement, even in those with higher measured IQs. Poor scholastic performance predicts both labour market disadvantage and poor mental health status in later life. Around 40 per cent of these children who complete their mandatory basic schooling fail to seek further training or regular employment, and the same figure become involved with the criminal justice system in adolescence (Jay and Padilla 1987; Wagner *et al*. 1993).

Of those recorded in clinical (rather than community samples), emotionally disturbed children have high levels of abuse or neglect in their family of origin, with estimates ranging from 20 per cent (Quinn and Epstein 1998) to 65 per cent (Zeigler-Dendy 1989). Quinn and Epstein (*ibid.*) also found that this family of origin population is disproportionately poor, with 40 per cent receiving welfare benefits and with only 60 per cent of fathers and less than 50 per cent of mothers being in employment. McLeod and Nonnemaker (2000) studied poor children and disaggregated racial and ethnic differences. They found that in white people, single mother status and prior maternal 'delinquency' predictably amplified poverty-derived stress on their children. In poor black people, low maternal self-esteem was more relevant in explaining this stress. In other words, long-term poverty increases the overall risk of psychological problems in children but individual and racial differences are also discernible

Given this picture of multiple disadvantage, what implications does having a mental health problem in childhood have for a developmental trajectory? Now, we turn to the link between childhood and adulthood emotional difficulties.

The importance of later childhood and adolescence

The bulk of the professional discussion about life-span and mental health emphasises *early* childhood (see the introduction). However, recently, more and more studies are emphasising the critical role of later childhood and adolescence. Longitudinal studies such as the 1970 British Birth Cohort Study (BCS) and the 1958 National Child Development Study (NCDS) have used repeated measures at different time points. Summarising the findings of the two cohort studies, Sacker *et al.* (1999) note:

- Neither direct health selection nor social causation fully explains the relationship between social class and mental health at 23 and 33 (NCDS) or 26 (BCS).
- Both psychological problems and lower paternal social class in adolescence increase the risk of mental health problems in adulthood (NCDS&BCS).
- Achieved social position in early adulthood is affected both by the father's social class and psychological problems in adolescence (NCDS&BCS).
- Approximately 50 per cent of the relationship between social class and mental health is accounted for by these pathways from paternal social class and adolescent problems by the age of 23 (NCDS) and 26 (BCS). By the age of 33 this relationship rises to nearly 100 per cent (NCDS).
- The continuation of behavioural problems in adulthood from adolescence is greater for men than women, and women show more intergenerational social mobility (NCDS&BCS) but intragenerational mobility is about the same in both sexes (NCDS).

Further evidence that later childhood and adolescence is important comes from longitudinal studies of conduct disorders in children and early onset psychosis. The Epidemiological Catchment Area study (Regier *etal.* 1988) found that the median age of onset of mental disorder was 16 years. Studies of conduct disorders show an interaction between concurrent family of origin features. Low parental social class, urban living, domestic violence and physical chastisement not only characterise the families of juvenile delinquents but go on to predict violent criminality in young adulthood. Teenagers with behavioural problems who persevere in their violent ways have abnormally high rates of childhood neglect and abuse (see above). In the USA, the National Institute of Justice found that the latter increase the risk of arrest as a juvenile by 50 per cent and arrest as an adult by 38 per cent and arrest for violent crime by 38 per cent (*Combating Violence and Delinquency* 1996).

The link between childhood and adult mental health status

Although the biological and environmental variants of the professional mental health literature we noted at the start of the chapter are discrepant, they can be reconciled by appeals to the biopsychosocial model. Such a model accepts that various levels of biological vulnerability coexist with pathogenic environmental and social events, which may be conceptualised as triggers or partial aetiological factors (Kendler 1998). Whether or not such a reconciliation is forged, the various theories we are offered about the genesis of mental health problems all agree on the existence of a developmental *trajectory*. That is, there is an implicit consensus across competing positions that a susceptibility to mental health problems in adult life is traceable to early life (at the stage of the embryo, the foetus, the infant or the young child). Even the literature on Post-Traumatic Stress Disorder (PTSD), which strongly emphasises contingent traumatic events, concedes some degree of individual vulnerability. How else can we account for the fact that people are affected to varying extents by the same traumatic events or adverse conditions?

In her review of 'early adversity and subsequent pathology', Widom (1998) makes the important point that childhood victimisation is rarely a one-off event but should be seen as part of a pathogenic system or milieu. This echoes a similar point made by Briere and Runtz (1987) when they discuss childhood sexual abuse, namely:

> Although symptomatology in adulthood may covary with early sexual abuse, in the absence of further data it is not clear whether the former is caused by the latter or whether both are actually a function of some third variable, such as dysfunctional family dynamics. (Briere and Runtz 1987: 51)

Children who are in abusive family systems are likely to suffer an uncaring environment before specifiable acts (of sexual contact or physical violence) emerge. For this reason, there is some conceptual cloudiness about the salient features which are relevant to reconstruct when tracing the pathogenic pathways from family events to immediate and subsequent mental health consequences. Put differently, whilst it is now very clear that early adversity has a negative impact on the well-being of children, immediately and later in their lives, at present it is less clear how causal pathways operate.

Whilst early abuse does not wholly explain the existence of adult mental health problems, compared to other explanations for mental ill-health its contribution is highly certain. Other aetiological 'candidates' favoured in partisan areas of the professional literature include genetic proneness to anxiety, depression or psychosis (from biological psychiatrists), attachment problems (from attachment theorists), inadequate defence mechanisms (from psychoanalysts) classical and operant conditioning (from behaviourists) and negative cognitive schemata (from cognitivists). Whilst these represent competing players on an unresolved aetiological field, childhood trauma has an incontestable pathogenic role in creating a *susceptibility* to a range of problems. It has a discernible impact on the mental health of both men (especially substance abuse) and women (especially anxiety and depression).

The gender differences suggest that post-traumatic symptom presentation is mediated by a developing gender identity during and subsequent to childhood victimisation. This may also account for gender differences in suicidal behaviour in young people, where males significantly outweigh females. Suicide at this stage of life is a nihilistic turning against the self. This can be found also in female parasuicidal behaviour and self-harm. Other suggestive indicators about violence as an outcome of abuse are the sex differences in criminal activity. Also, men predominate in mentally disordered offender facilities. It is likely that distress is expressed more through violent and other antisocial acts by traumatised men, whereas women are more likely to present with psychiatric difficulties.

The work of George Brown and his colleagues has firmly illuminated pathways into depression for women. Within the model, susceptibility is acknowledged from two sources (biological predisposition and childhood vulnerability factors). Brown's model operates within a Durkheimian tradition and so includes its strengths and weaknesses. In terms of interactive causal pathways, Brown's model is consistent with an open systems model of interacting multiple variables operating at a moment in time (synchronic factors) and across time (diachronic factors). The inclusive emphasis upon material events and subjective factors is a clear strength. However, it has no framework for analysing the epistemological status of categories such as 'depression'. The validity of the latter diagnosis is explicitly accepted in the early pages of *The Social Origins of Depression* (Brown and Harris 1978). The concept of depression has been critically appraised by both poststructuralists (Parker *et al.* 1997) and critical realists (Pilgrim and Bentall 1998). Also, Brown's model has nothing firmly to say about men.

Service contact and social disadvantage during adolescence

There is a growing literature on the impact of therapeutic interventions on troubled children and teenagers (Buchanan 1999). The role of schools is also significant in this regard.[1] Influences on what encourages or discourages help-seeking is relevant to whether or not young people experiencing emotional distress access support. Potentially, the latter may help reduce the risk of mental health problems continuing into adulthood and of low school attainment leading to enduring socio-economic disadvantage. The reluctance to seek help amongst adolescents has been the subject of studies which focus on individual characteristics and service contact.[2] Whilst such individualistic factors are likely to be relevant, the perception of services (as being non-stigmatising and appropriate) will also influence help-seeking in vulnerable young people, in a way that may help their life-chances.

There is evidence of a reluctance of young people to engage with conventional health services (Kari *et al.* 1997) and a relatively underdeveloped system within schools (Daniels *et al.* 1999). More-over, the possibility remains of a relatively unexplored association between perceptions of coercion and help-seeking. As we have seen in Chapter 3, this is evident in conventional health services, even in primary care. The fact that behavioural problems are associated with exclusion and other enforced social sanctions may also affect the willingness of young people to access support from official agencies. School-based support services could be the basis of problem solving and might pre-empt the need for exclusion (particularly those based on peer group interventions). Nonetheless, the coercion and stigma associated with service provision currently made available or imposed on young people are likely to continue to be implicated in a cycle of inequality.

Social integration in adulthood

If the above section indicates that adverse conditions in early years of life (plus genetic and congenital loading) are the foundations of inequalities in mental health status, life events and other stressors during adulthood are also relevant. If a benign and secure family context is a protective factor in childhood, then triggering and buf-fering factors which are a function of social integration and victimisa-tion in adulthood also need to be considered. We deal with the issue of victimisation in Chapter 6: here we deal with social integration.

Durkheim's classic study of suicide noted that individuals who were poorly integrated were at an increased risk but so, too, were those who were overintegrated. This suggests that in adulthood, probably more than in childhood, a social and interpersonal milieu which might be optimal for mental health has to offer opportunities for autonomy whilst also demanding and rewarding social cohesion and conformity. An adult in any culture needs to feel a sense of belonging but must also feel that their autonomy and privacy (their 'personhood') are respected. A number of disruptions to this balance can occur during adult life at work and in domestic contexts. Moreover, material inequality has direct and indirect effects on mental health in both settings (Fryer 1995) suggesting that insults to personhood are created, or amplified, by conditions of poverty or relative deprivation. Below we consider socio-economic and psycho-logical adversity in adulthood under three headings reflecting aspects of social integration: the negative impact of labour market disadvantage; homelessness; and intimacy and separation. These three aspects have a particular salience in middle adulthood when work (as a right or obligation) is a role expectation. At this stage in the life course, the formation and maintenance of relationships brings with it particular psychosocial challenges. As for homelessness, although this might affect people of all ages, those of working age who have no shelter have become a controversial focus in mental health debates and so we offer a brief commentary on the topic.

The negative impact of labour market disadvantage

Unemployment may potentially lead to four economic outcomes. The first is of economic advantage (inherited money leading to the freedom to abandon the work role; an advantageous retirement package etc.). The second is one of financial *status quo*. An example here is where only low paid work is available, so that a person on welfare payments is little or no better off when working. The third is one of relative poverty – unemployment leads to dependency on State payments, which ensure a subsistence lifestyle. Fourth, in countries where there is no welfare 'safety net' an unemployed person may be able to afford no food or shelter and so lives in absolute poverty.

It is obvious that each of these possibilities has different psychosocial implications. The first may (though not inevitably) lead to improvements in mental health. The second indicates personal stagnation or that any slight deterioration in income conditions will probably lead to multiple loss (of buying power, social status, structured daily activity and self-esteem). The third is the likelihood of chronic economic adversity. Here, the existential challenge is not of tolerating loss but of surviving permanent social exclusion. The fourth possibility occurs on the margins of developed societies in homeless populations but is more prevalent in less developed countries (see below). When absolute poverty is experienced, then physical survival, not just psychological well-being, is at stake.

However, these possible outcomes are not neatly boundaried for all cases. For example, the lottery millionaire of the first scenario may experience some of the losses in the second. Also, those with chronic low pay may be propelled into absolute poverty. Patel (2001) draws attention to the experience of subsistence farmers in India who lost crops in the monsoon season failures of the mid-1990s. Their low harvests led them to choose between starvation or bonded labour to money lenders. Suicide rates leapt in this population during this period.

These complex and overlapping outcomes are rehearsed here to highlight that simplistic questions, such as 'does unemployment cause mental ill-health?', need to be answered with reference to a network of political and psychosocial mediating factors. Was the person forced to leave work? Are they chronically or intermittently outside the labour market? How much does a particular nation-state ensure that its poorest population stratum does not fall into absolute poverty? Also, as we will see later, employment brings with it a set of stressors and so is not a wholly benign alternative trajectory for those of working age. Those in scenarios three and four are also more likely to be poorly nourished and live in stressful localities. Their physical health is adversely affected, which may have an indirect impact on experienced well-being (see Chapter 3).

With these provisos in mind, what do we know about the impact of unemployment on mental health? Kasl *et al.* (1998) in their review of the topic point out that we can argue with some certainty that, overall, unemployment has a negative impact on mental health. This broad conclusion holds true for community surveys of so-called 'sub-clinical' decrements in well-being (mainly depressive symptomatology). However, it is more difficult to justify from the studies available that unemployment has a clear and predictable causal effect on other adverse mental health outcomes (once depressive symptoms are excluded).

Longitudinal studies looking at the impact of re-employment consistently demonstrate an improvement in mental health scores, but becoming (and remaining) unemployed introduces a question about the *direction* of causality (the selection versus causation debate). Also, unemployment is a state to which individuals may habituate, whereas insecure and stressful employment may create enduring psychological instability (see later). Consequently, it cannot be taken for granted that losing employment always represents a shift from a secure to a less secure existential state.

Turning to the ambiguous or reciprocal relationship between labour market disadvantage and those with a diagnosed mental illness, the two are certainly correlated, even if the direction of causality is ambiguous in particular cases. In Britain, those recorded with a diagnosis of neurosis, compared to the general population, are four to five times more likely to be unemployed, twice as likely to be receiving income support and four to five times more likely to be receiving invalidity benefits. Patients with a diagnosis of psychosis only have a one in four chance of being in employment (Jenkins and Singh 2001).

The outcome of those experiencing psychotic disorders is affected by employment status – those chronically unemployed are more likely to relapse than those entering or re-entering the labour market (Warner 1984). Thus, whilst labour market disadvantage may cause mental ill-health, psychiatric patients are definitely more likely than others to be unemployed. Moreover, re-employment is a crucial recovery factor in those with psychotic episodes.

The relationship of labour market disadvantage and mental health is also characterised by cohort effects – life-span effects are not recycled evenly from one generation to another. For example, during periods of high employment, those of working age will be buffered from the stress of insecure employment more than those in periods of economic depression (Pearlin and Scaff 1996) and those with pre-existing mental health problems will find it easier to find work and thus enjoy the recovery effects of social reintegration (Warner 1984).

Because macro-economic conditions vary over time, and thus affect age cohorts differentially, Cahill (1983) argued that the relationship between labour market disadvantage and mental health has to be considered in relation to the dynamic relationship between five contemporary socio-economic features: instability in the business cycle; unemployment; inequality in income distribution; capital mobility; and fragmentation of the work process. Kasl *et al.* (1998), summarising this complex open system picture, comment:

> In short, job loss as an acute event and unemployment as a particularly enduring exposure are both richly embedded in a social matrix involving the interdependence of the individual, the family, the network of friends and relatives, the immediate community, the regional economy, and society as a whole. This leaves ample room for variability of impact, linked to variations in the meaning of the experience and to the role of diverse moderators that affect the processes and the outcomes. (Kasl *et al.* 1998: 112)

A labour process emphasis has been augmented by more recent commentaries on consumption. In the past twenty years, North

American and European societies have witnessed an increasing emphasis upon identity being defined by consumer behaviour, especially in younger people. This has led some to note an age-related profile of anxiety in the life-span in modern society, with young adults being more prone to debt-induced anxiety (Drentea 2000). The importance of cohort effects is dramatically demonstrated by the paradox of the raised post-Second World War incidence of diagnosed mental disorder in young people in developed societies, despite contemporary evidence of improved physical health. Some of this increase may be linked to increased illicit drug and alcohol use and the decline in the socially integrative role of religious affiliation.

Taken together, the above studies indicate that unemployment shapes mental health outcomes in complex ways. Some of these shaping factors are positive some of the time. However, most shaping factors are negative: objective and subjective losses; chronic socio-economic adversity; absolute as well as relative poverty; and the indirect effects of poor nutrition, inferior physical health and raised levels of local environmental stressors. These are compounded by those with mental health problems tending to have: relative low levels of cultural capital (poorer education); painful biographical baggage (higher rates of neglect and abuse in childhood); and weaker social networks in localities, which themselves have low levels of social capital.

This adverse picture is aggravated by the primary disability of mental health problems and their amplification by the stigma and social rejection expressed by neighbours. Thus, once a person is both unemployed *and* has a mental health problem, they are caught in a 'ball of wax' of reciprocally reinforcing adverse factors. We return to this ball of wax phenomenon in poor localities in Chapter 6.

Employment status and mental health – a complex relationship

The above discussion of unemployment might imply that employment is linked to mental health maintenance or gain. However, there are mixed conditions, and thus effects, in sub-populations of the labour market. For example, some types of work expose employees to an increased risk of trauma (e.g., the emergency services and the armed forces), whilst others are noteworthy for repetitive tedium (e.g., conveyer-belt factory work) or low task control (those at the base of a hierarchy) or job insecurity (those on temporary contracts). Work which is prone to job insecurity and career stagnation brings with it low morale (Burchell 1992). Thus, employment status is relatively easy to study if a dichotomy (employed/not employed) is deployed, but the results of such investigations are consequently limited by the likely existence of graduated effects operating along a continuum of employment (see below), which contains different forms of occupational stress, frustration and loss.

Whilst there is a consistent picture in the cross-sectional studies that labour market disadvantage is linked to raised levels of both stress and mental illness, an interpretive difficulty relates to the direction of causality. Does the stress of unemployment and poor employment lead to distress? Alternatively, might psychologically vulnerable individuals be unable to cope with permanent work? This conundrum is a rephrasing of the social selection versus social causation debate. Longitudinal studies resolve the problem to some degree. Dooley *et al.* (2000) used such an approach to investigate 'underemployment'. This preferred construct is operationalised by them as a continuum from fulfilling well-paid work ('adequate employment') to low-status work, which might be involuntary or part-time and is ill-paid ('inadequate employment'). The authors tracked more than 5000 young people in the US who were adequately employed in 1992 for two years. They found that, controlling for prior depression, raised levels of newly diagnosed depression were discernible *both* in those who became unemployed *and* in those who shifted to lower status and pay. They also found that other variables might buffer or amplify mental health problems in those with a negatively shifted employment status. Marriage mitigated the stress of the adverse shift, whereas poor education and low job satisfaction amplified the risk of depression.

The above picture was also found in an Australian study (Graetz 1993), which compared satisfied and dissatisfied workers and unemployed people. Satisfied workers had the highest mental health scores, dissatisfied the lowest, with the unemployed sample scoring in between. What low-paid and unemployed people have in common is the struggle to survive long-term financial strain – debt, 'making ends meet' and being able to afford holidays and other stress-reducing leisure activities. They also often contend with 'neighbourhood strain' (see below). Also, being in work may be a buffer against life events, with evidence that unemployed people are more susceptible to symptom formation in their wake (Kessler *et al.* 1987).

The interacting variables of type of employment and adequacy, educational level and marital status highlight a key point about differential vulnerability to mental health problems in adulthood. Trajectories of mental health are not linked to labour market position *per se* but seemingly to a person's *total experience of social integration or exclusion and their own sense of robustness or vulnerability*. This existential state has multiple objective indicators (close confiding relationships, structured daily activity, access to safety, privacy, leisure activity, etc.) and a single but shifting subjective indicator (an adult's view of themselves and their relationship to others – their self-identity). The shifting experience is determined by one fixed and predictable variable (ageing) operating in a multi-factorial open system of the type described by Brown and his colleagues (life events, educational status, marital status, loss of significant others, etc.). The latter effects on mental health might be negative (e.g., loss) or positive (e.g., new educational opportunities).

Another open system variable is spatial. Low-income people can only afford to live in poor neighbourhoods. Ross (2000) studied a 2482 sample from the 1995 Community Crime and Health Survey of Illinois and found that controlling for other variables, about 50 per cent of the variance of stress-related depression in poor neighbourhoods was linked to the direct impact of poverty (financial strain and life-chance and activity restriction). The rest was accounted for by the cultural impact of the quality of life in such localities, which is driven down by high crime rates, noise, litter, graffiti, vandalism, visible effects of illicit drug use and tense relationships. In these localities, social cohesion (or informal social control) is eroded and this becomes a constant background stressor for inhabitants. The converse of this is evident in the neighbourhoods inhabited by high earners, which tend to be quiet, and relatively free of litter, crime, traffic and noise ('leafy suburbs').

Whilst depression rates tend to rise in poor neighbourhoods, not all residents are depressed despite a backdrop for all residents of low levels of social capital. This points us towards some individual or biographical effects, such as the presence or absence of childhood abuse and individual cognitive differences in learned coping strategies. Also, caution needs to be applied about overstating the ecological factor, or reducing explanations of mental ill-health to contemporary environmental stressors – the 'ecological fallacy'. For example, in densely populated capital cities such as London, rich people and poor people live in close proximity. Thus, neighbourhood cannot automatically be taken as a proxy for SES. As noted earlier, SES differences exist in mental health scores but vary from locality to locality.

Taken as a whole, the literature on unemployment and employment suggests the following:

- Broadly, those in work enjoy better mental health than those out of work. This conclusion is confirmed by sequential studies of unemployed and re-employed samples.
- However, unemployed and employed populations produce overlapping, not discrete, distributions of mental health scores. Inadequately employed people tend to have poorer mental health scores than those who are unemployed.
- Although the direction of causality remains ambiguous about the correlation between severe mental health problems and labour market disadvantage, psychiatric patients are more likely to be excluded from work than non-patients and their prognosis is improved by occupational reintegration.
- Whereas depressive symptoms are a sensitive indicator of labour market effects, this is not the case with other forms of diagnosis. As far as anxiety states and psychosis are concerned, labour market disadvantage is apparent. However, this could be accounted for by a primary disability, rendering patients unfit to work, and the compounding effects of employment discrimination and public stigma. This raises questions about the direction of causality between many mental health problems and employment status.
- Being in work may be tedious, entail poor task control and it may be insecure. These conditions of 'inadequate employment' create a negative impact on the mental health of the one stratum of the workforce.
- The chances of *particular* unemployed or inadequately employed individuals suffering mental health problems are shaped by factors other than just their employment status. In particular, for some symptoms there are age cohort effects (younger workers being more vulnerable), as well as the impact of isolation or intimacy and the sustaining effects of cultural capital based upon high educational levels. Locality is important, as is the pre-existing level of psychological robustness of the person suffering labour market disadvantage. Social support and access

to leisure activities mediate mental health status in those unemployed or inadequately employed.

Homelessness

Access to regular shelter and sustenance defines the boundary between relative and absolute poverty. Consequently, homeless populations represent the poorest of the poor in developed societies. They are subject to forms and degrees of stress which are found less, or not at all, in those with homes. In particular, homeless people are 'disaffiliated', that is, they lack regular forms of social support present in other social groups, even those with low incomes. Depression in homeless groups is mediated by a number of factors including educational level, length of time homeless, daily hassles, physical health problems, life events and prior psychiatric hospitalisation (Gory *et al.* 1990). However, although homelessness is depressogenic, as we note below, homeless people are not more likely than other poor groups to be diagnosed as being mentally ill. Indeed, prevalence rates of depression are higher in the housed poor. The homeless are more likely to have other personal difficulties however.

The social problem of homelessness has become entwined with mental health problems in the professional literature in a number of ways. It has been a focus for those who fought a rearguard action against mental hospital closure (arguing that ex-residents would find themselves on the streets). It has also been a point of debate about the direction of causality between mental health problems and homelessness. A recent summary of the US literature shows that there is no doubt that prevalence rates for psychiatric diagnoses of psychosis and substance abuse are significantly higher in homeless populations compared to those in regular housing.

Homelessness is a politically controversial issue in developed countries for reasons other than its ambiguous relationship with mental health problems. During the 1990s, the richest country in the world, the USA, had estimated rates of around 8 per cent lifetime prevalence of homelessness (Link *et al.* 1994). However, lower rates than this were insistently claimed by conservative politicians. Part of this political debate relates to causality. Conservative commentators express a view based upon individualism – homelessness is a product of the aggregate of individual fecklessness and/or personal deficits or defects (such as mental illness). More left-leaning protagonists argue the reverse – that the socio-economic adversity inherent in homelessness is a context in which mental health problems arise.

Studies which have disaggregated the effects of poverty from homeless status indicate that the latter group are more likely to abuse illicit drugs and alcohol but do not have higher rates of mental illness than the housed poor (Toro 1998). Even this disaggregation does not define the direction of causality or distinguish causes from consequences. Ultimately, the question of causality is impossible to pin down clearly because subjects cannot be randomly assigned to experimental groups.

Longitudinal naturalistic studies are currently under way and Toro (*ibid.*) examines the first indications of what can and cannot be said about the relationship between homelessness and mental health problems. After reviewing the evidence, he rejects an emphasis upon deinstitutionalisation – most of the people with mental health problems who are homeless are young and were never institutionalised. In most developed countries, deinstitutionalisation led to the systematic State-monitored resettlement of ex-hospital residents.

Substance abuse seems to predict homelessness (with or without the presence of mental health problems). Studies in different countries have revealed a consistent pattern of raised levels of substance abuse in the homeless, with cross-national estimates of prevalence varying from 25–50 per cent in women and from 50–75 per cent in men (Teeson *et al.* 2000). As we indicate in Chapter 6, when discussing violence, the interaction of psychosis and substance abuse may define a particularly vulnerable group of people. They are vulnerable to self-neglect, self-harm and are more likely to be hostile to others. Toro also concludes that past family violence also increases the probability of a person becoming homeless.

Homeless patients do seem to have a different symptom profile to domiciled poor patients in contact with mental health services. The former are more likely to be substance abusers and meet criteria for antisocial personality disorder and are less likely to be depressed than the latter (North *et al.* 1997). When psychotic patients are compared, homeless people are more likely than domiciled comparisons to have had a criminal history, childhood conduct disorders and dysfunctional relationships with parents (including abuse), as well as having higher rates of substance misuse (Odell and Commander 2000; Sullivan *et al.* 2000).

Homelessness is a practical expression of extreme poverty. This obvious point is worth restating (see above discussion of unemployment). Although homeless people have some differentiating features from the 'housed poor', they still are, unambiguously, poor. Consequently, the adverse effects of poverty on mental health are important in homeless populations, as are the indirect effects of poor physical health. The latter is discussed later in relation to older people.

The literature from homelessness and mental health reflects some of the unresolved debates we noted in Chapter 1 about social drift and social causation. A major problem with the social psychiatric studies we cite here is the overemphasis on diagnosis in epidemiology and the underemphasis on biographical aspects. As we noted in Chapter 2, the work of Macintyre and others studying physical health demonstrates how a fine-grained experiential approach to studying the relationship between housing status and experienced well-being is important. Currently this importance has not been recognised by mainstream psychiatric epidemiology. This points up how a biosocial approach in psychiatry inevitably fails to address the experience of the people it studies.

Intimacy and separation

There is little evidence that the mental health impact of separation is linked to sexuality (see Chapter 6) but in the case of heterosexual couples there is a much higher incidence of a third party impact (upon offspring). Also, the data on divorce is methodologically more robust because it is a formally recorded social administrative category, which can be used to map mental health changes. Studies of separation in unmarried pairs (heterosexual or homosexual) is more difficult to investigate.

Bruce (1998) notes divorce itself may appear to be a discrete event but it is ambiguous when studying mental health impact. First, it is usually the culmination of a stressful process or a strained relationship over time. Second, mental health problems may be a cause, as well as a consequence, of divorce. Third, effects on mental health on the separating adults can be both direct and indirect, as well as affecting the mental health status of any children from the relationship.

Whilst higher rates of mental health problems are correlated with separation, the direction of causality is difficult to trace. Moreover, it is possible that confounding variables might account for both. Bruce (*ibid.*) gives the example of job loss. This stressor may increase marital stress *and* provoke depression or alcohol abuse. Bruce concludes that linear causal relationships cannot be deduced and that it may be wiser to think in terms of circular interactions and confounding variables.

If the data on the impact of separation on the adult parties is ambiguous, that on the offspring of splitting relationships is not. There are raised levels of dysfunctional states reported in the literature compared to non-divorced offspring, including conduct disorders, delinquency, personality disorders, anxiety states and depression (Dadds *et al.* 1992; Mann *et al.* 1990; Porter and O'Leary 1980; Stolberg *et al.* 1998). Post-divorced life brings with it an absence of a coordinated parental alliance in child rearing action, a disruption in the child's social network and may entail having to move house and school. An additional burden may be a reduced income available to support the child, if the non-custodial parent provides insufficient financial maintenance.

The actual legal event of divorce tends to have little or no immediate impact upon children or parents. The relevant impactful factors are pre-separation strain and the post-separation alterations in family life just noted. The impact during childhood of divorce is indicated by service involvement, with almost half of children in contact with mental health services coming from divorced families (a third of the married population) (Stolberg *et al.* 1998).

If separation negatively affects mental health, it generally holds that those currently married report greater well-being than those separated or widowed (with this effect being more prominent in men than women). In other words, single status is negatively correlated with mental health. However, those who are repeatedly married (after divorce or widowhood) accrue less and less mental health benefit from stable intimacy over time (Barrett 2000). The direction of causality is ambiguous – sequential relationships bring with them a sequence of losses, with anxiety and depression coming in their wake. However, those with mental health problems may have difficulties in sustaining intimate relationships, which could also account for Barrett's findings.

Finally, it is worth noting in this section that intimacy potentially brings with it risks not just benefits. We discuss this further in

Chapter 6 when summarising findings on domestic violence. Despite the latter, those in intimate relationships tend to fare better mental health-wise than those living alone.

Mental health and ageing

Until quite recently, it was a common cultural assumption that middle age was a significantly vulnerable phase of life. However, estimates of generalised distress are higher in childhood, young adulthood and very old age. Very broadly, there is a U-shaped relationship between age and distress. Within this U-shaped relationship, the incidence of depression is at its *lowest* in mid-life with the 'optimum' age of mental health averaging at 63 years (Wade and Cairney 1997). Even in the very old (80 years plus), mental health remains superior to that of early adulthood in developed countries. This may in part be due to lowering expectations with age and the rawness of adverse childhood experiences in adolescence and young adulthood during a challenging transitional life phase.

Older people are more prone to biological conditions, which affect mental health, than are younger adults. The most obvious example of this is dementia, which has a variety of causes, some of which (e.g., in arterio-sclerotic dementia) are better understood than others (e.g., in Alzheimer's Disease) (Cooper 1989). However, older people are more likely to be diagnosed with depression than with dementia – a point we will explore later. Because dementia is a deteriorating condition but depression is reversible or episodic, the prevalence to incidence ratio of the former is greater than the latter.

In Western countries, which have seen a recent increase in older populations, the prevalence of dementia is set to increase. For example, in the UK it was estimated in 1992 that the prevalence of dementia would rise over a twenty-five-year period from 500,000 to 750,000 (Alzheimer's Disease Report 1992). The prevalence rate of dementia in those between 65 and 75 years of age is only around 1 per cent. However, this rises to 10 per cent after 75 years, and by 85 years of age nearly 50 per cent of the population is deemed to be dementing (Satlin *et al.* 1999).

Elsewhere (Pilgrim and Rogers 1999), we have noted that mental health problems in old age can be accounted for by a set of interacting biological, psychological and social factors, which we summarise below. Before doing this, it is worth noting an overriding vulnerability factor – displacement from the labour market. This has two consequences. First, older people tend to have a reduced income. The population-level consequence of this is that those with low socioeconomic status in the middle years may become significantly poor in old age. In the other direction, those with greater economic resources in their middle years are in a position to plan for retirement and make investments to cushion their salary loss. Those in stable high status jobs are likely to have good industrial pensions. Those in low status and intermittent employment are more likely to be reliant on a residual state pension. Those who have been chronically unemployed will remain unemployed but will also have to deal with other conditions of adversity which come with this status (such as an increased risk of physical health problems). Thus, as with the points made above about poverty during the years of employment, material adversity may play a part in affecting the mental health of low socio-economic status elders.

The second point about the unemployed status of older people is that financial security may combine with the removal of the stress of higher-status employees to create mental health *gain* after retirement. This appears to be the implication of the research reported by Blaxter (1990) on self-reports of well-being over time. On average, the rich seem to get richer as far as mental health is concerned, with those in social classes 1 and 2 significantly improving with age and those in classes 4 and 5 deteriorating. Similarly, Murphy (1982) found that material adversity, defined by recent housing and income problems, was significantly correlated with depression in old age. A further complicating factor is that whilst retirement is a culturally expected life transition, it may be imposed on some people prematurely by illness or redundancy. This dislocation may be traumatic or demoralising because of role and status loss and imposed relative poverty.

As we noted earlier, studies of depression suggest that there is a U-shaped relationship in adulthood until death, with middle-aged people being less depressed than older old people and young adults (Kessler *et al.* 1992; Mirowsky and Reynolds 2000). Schieman *et al.* (2001) used data from the US General Social Surveys in 1996 and 1998 to disaggregate particular influences in this pattern. They found that low education and widowhood contribute to raised levels of depression in older people, but some elders are not more depressed as they age because of less time demands and greater financial resources (confirming the finding of Blaxter noted earlier). In mid-life, decreased rates of depression are linked to religious affiliation but increased rates are found in those suffering physical ill-health.

With this backdrop of socio-economic and cultural influences which may improve or aggravate mental health status with age in mind, we now turn to a further examination of biological, psychological and social effects.

- *Biological factors* – Both dementia and depression have underlying biological influences. Decreasing cardio-vascular efficiency during the life-span increases the chances of multiple vessel ruptures in the brain, which can create a dementing process. This type of dementia is a function of cortical strokes, or multi-infarct disease, which increase in probability in those with chronic hypertension and/or diabetes. Although the aetiology of the non-arterio-sclerotic dementias may be still contested, post-mortem examination reveals extensive brain damage in those suffering from Pick's Disease and Alzheimer's Disease. However, occasionally brain disease is not evident post-mortem, despite clear cognitive deficits pathognomic of dementia (Kitwood 1988). In strict logical terms, 'dementia' describes a group of *neurological* diseases, or symptoms linked to other degenerative physical conditions such as Huntingdon's Disease or Parkinson's Disease. (Around 30 per cent of older people with Parkinson's Disease show signs of dementia.) The classification of dementia as an 'organic mental illness' was historically based upon its functional symptoms, which are mainly about the role failure and rule breaking following from memory loss, disorientation, aphasia, agnosia and other cognitive deficits. Consequently, 'dements' (cf. 'aments', now those with a learning disability) was a general social administrative category of madness, defined by a loss of reason from any cause, which was managed in the Victorian asylum system. Depression, a 'functional mental illness', is biologically influenced in a different way. With age, there is an increased probability of severe and multiple physical illnesses. With this, comes functional loss and chronic pain, which are misery-inducing (Brayne and Ames 1988). In one study of 100 patients referred over a 30-month period to a psychogeriatric service (Dover and McWilliam 1992), only 3 per cent of the men and 20 per cent of the women were found to be physically well. Only one in five older inpatients with physical illnesses recover from depressed mood before death (Cole and Bellevance 1997). Around a third of those with dementia are also depressed (Satlin *et al*. 1999). Thus, mental health problems in old age are commonly associated with physical co-morbidity.

- *Psychological factors* – The loss of significant others and physical function is not limited to old age (it is fairly common in middle age as well) but later life brings with it an *aggregating* experience of loss. In old age, not only are parents usually dead but so are more and more peers and some old people may be unfortunate enough to outlive their adult children. As for spouses, it is rare for couples to die together, which leaves widows (and less often widowers) as a significant feature of older populations. Not only does single and multiple bereavement increase the probability of diagnosable depression in community samples, it also raises the general probability of illness and help-seeking (Clayton 1998). Clayton (1986) reported statistically significant differences between bereaved and non-bereaved controls in relation to abdominal pain, alcohol and psychotropic drug use and arthritic pain. Widowers are at increased risk of death within the first six months of losing their spouse but this mortality link is not consistently reported in studies examining widows (Clayton 1998). Even in the odd study, which fails to show an immediate increase in the bereaved male mortality rate, an increase in cirrhosis of the liver culminating in premature death is still demonstrated (Helsing *et al*. 1982). Apart from cirrhosis, alcohol abuse in bereavement leads to a loss of self-respect, as well as the debilitating experience of a chronic toxic reaction. These feed into, and partially define, a depressive episode. Thus, a psychosomatic interface is clearly apparent during bereavement, taking us back to the previous point about the biological influence upon depression.
- *Social factors* – We have already emphasised the economic impact of poverty in older people. In addition, a practical consequence of aggregating loss may be a restricted social network and an increased risk of personal isolation. This process may be amplified by episodes of physical illness or chronic disability affecting mobility or sensory acuity. Studies of community samples of older people demonstrate that close confiding relationships are

a protective factor against depression (Lowenthal 1965; Murphy 1982), echoing the findings of Brown and Harris, discussed earlier, about a younger sample. For those who enter care, a known home is lost (both objectively and subjectively) and the new environment may be understimulating and not 'homely'. Indeed, low mood is such a common feature of residential care that psychiatrists find it difficult to distinguish common dysthymia in these settings from 'clinical depression' (Murphy 1982). Findings in different countries show depression rates of between 30 per cent and 40 per cent in older people in residential facilities (Mann *et al.* 1984; Snowden and Donnelly 1986; Spagnoli *et al.* 1986). Community surveys in a variety of countries in the 1980s demonstrated depression rates in non-institutionalised elders of between 5 per cent (Maule *et al.* 1984) and 26 per cent (Kay *et al.* 1964), with typical rates of between 11 per cent and 15 per cent in the UK (Copeland *et al.* 1987) and 8 per cent–15 per cent in the USA (Blazer 1994). Thus, even in non-residential settings, diagnosable depression is not uncommon in old age. Another social factor to consider is that of the power relationship entailed in caring for older people. As with children, this can lead to abuse. A review of the Scandinavian literature found rates of elder abuse of between 8 per cent and 17 per cent (Hydle 1993). Paveza *et al.* (1992) found that within a year of a diagnosis of Alzheimer's Disease, 5.4 per cent of lay carers were violent to their relative. However, 15.8 per cent of sufferers were also violent, indicating the risk of an aggressive spiral in dementia care. Finally in this section, Kitwood and his colleagues (Kitwood 1997; Kitwood and Bredin 1992) have emphasised the relevance of social factors in dementia outcomes. They argue that a medical approach to dementia leads to an overemphasis on the disease and not the person, generating a malignant social-psychological field in which the dementing person is lost and their personhood obscured. This leads to a socially derived amplification of the dementing process.

It is clear that the mental health of older people has to be understood in multifactorial terms, entailing complex interactions between biological, psychological and social factors. Adversity can be seen as intrinsic to old age (biological decline and psychological loss) but the mental health impact of this intrinsic trend is mediated by social factors and the degree of psychological robustness inherited from earlier years. Social determinants include economic status, the retention or provision of upportive social networks and the presence of benign rather than abusive carers.

Mental health inequality in later life, as in younger years, is thus a function of socio-economic status, life events, personality and inter-personal factors, especially the presence of support networks. How-ever, the co-presence of physical illness is much more common than in younger people with mental health problems. As a consequence, the class-predicted effects of *physical morbidity* in old age need to be brought in as an indirect manifestation of social inequality in those with mental health problems. This indirect sign of physical health inequalities adds to the direct impact of poverty upon depressed mood in elders. The poor older person is at significant increased risk of physical and mental health problems both separately and in combination.

Conclusion

This chapter has highlighted that inequality can be thought of in a longitudinal, as well as cross-sectional, way. In the language of general systems theory, it is about 'diachronic' (across time) not just 'synchronic' (moment in time) features. From conception and before birth, we are unequal – our genetic material and uterine envir-onment are not a 'level playing field'. The foetus in the womb of an opiate or alcohol addict is already disadvantaged. The *amount* of variance in later mental health status attributable to ante-natal life remains contested but it is clearly relevant. When we shift to the quality of childhood experience, only the most dogmatic genetic determinist would challenge its causal or dispositional relevance, especially in relation to the strong evidence about the immediate and long-term mental health impact of neglect and abuse.

Trajectories of poor mental health are discernible but they have to be understood in multifactorial terms. Each phase of the life-span includes relevant 'constants' across time – good physical health, high socio-economic status, benign/supportive personal relationships and positive coping strategies all predict and constitute good mental health. However, the relevant salience of these varies over time. In childhood, secure attachment is particularly important. For those of working age, the balance between social conformity and personal autonomy is crucial. In the very old, physical health status takes on a greater relevance for mental health.

These different considerations along the life-span are associated with different emphases in professional knowledge. For example, the bio-psychosocial model seems to be most persuasive in relation to older people. By contrast, those emphasising a social causation model are on their strongest grounds in relation to adults of working age. Socially derived stress is unequivocally implicated in explaining depression at this life stage. Also, even in those who are psychotic, where primary causation is multifactorial, opportunities for social integration significantly affect prognosis or recovery. It is in childhood that we find the greatest tension in professional accounts. As we noted in the introduction, so many models (genetic, congenital, psychodynamic, behavioural, cognitive) vie for pre-eminence in explaining childhood disorders and the role of early life in explaining current and later vulnerability to mental health problems.

6

Violence: victimhood and discrimination

Introduction

This chapter has an overarching aim of providing a balanced exploration of the relationship between mental health and violence. This can be contrasted with the narrow and often prejudicially driven view to be found in media reporting and political populism. It is important, by way of introduction, to signal the broader prejudicial and discriminatory character of our current dominant political discourse, which emphasises the relationship between mental health problems and dangerousness.

We have noted elsewhere (Pilgrim and Rogers 1999) that judgements about, and penalties for, actual or perceived dangerousness in different types of social group are not consistent. We demonstrate this point by the use of Table 6.1.

The rules applying to the detention of psychiatric patients are more Draconian than for other groups. Detention is without trial other than for mentally disordered offenders and, even in the case of the latter, detention is open-ended, not defined in advance (cf. prisoners). This discriminatory treatment of psychiatric patients was pointed up by Thomas Szasz:

> Drunken drivers are dangerous both to themselves and to others. They injure and kill many more people than, for example, persons with paranoid delusions of persecution. Yet people labeled 'paranoid' are readily committable, while drunken drivers are not ... Some types of dangerous behaviour are even rewarded. Racecar drivers, trapeze artists, and astronauts receive admiration and applause ... Thus it is not dangerousness in general that is at issue here, but rather the manner in which one is dangerous. (Szsaz 1963: 46).

Table 6.1   Mental health and dangerousness

	Law breaker		Law abiding		Law breaker		Law abiding	
	Sick Detained	Free	Detained	Free	Well Detained	Free	Detained	Free
Dangerous	1	2	3	4	5	6	7	8
Non-dangerous	9	10	11	12	13	14	15	16

Cell 1:   Mentally disordered offenders
Cell 2:   Mentally disordered offenders prior to detection
Cell 3:   Civil compulsory admissions to psychiatric hospitals
Cell 4:   People who are HIV + who indulge in unprotected sexual intercourse
Cell 5:   Convicted prisoners
Cell 6:   Drunken/speeding car drivers
Cell 7:   Prisoners of war
Cell 8:   Members of the SAS
Cell 9:   Petty criminal prisoners who are psychologically disturbed
Cell 10:   Petty criminals on probation
Cell 11:   Old people forcibly hospitalised under the 1948 National Assistance Act because they live in insanitary conditions
Cell 12:   People in the community who are depressed
Cell 13:   Prisoners guilty of 'white collar' crimes such as fraud
Cell 14:   Un-apprehended shoplifters
Cell 15:   Victims of child abuse who are taken into care
Cell 16:   The assumed societal norm

It is this question about 'the manner in which one is dangerous', as well as who is the agent of dangerous acts, which links the first and second halves of this chapter. Before returning in the second half to the issue of patient dangerousness, in the first half we address a common silence in political debates – the significance of violence in *generating* distress and dysfunction in many people with a psychiatric diagnosis. The irony of this relative silence is that psychiatric knowledge has been shaped often by a social context of warfare, which, *ipso facto*, has been dominated by violence.

Recently, violence has been viewed by Wilkinson (2000) as an integral part of interactions in society and an intelligible response to inequality and an uneven distribution of trust. In contrast to this normalised view of violence in unequal *social* relationships, the discussion of violence in relation to mental health is virtually always framed in terms of *individual* pathology. An approach to understanding mental health problems, which focuses on social processes characterised by violence, reframes individual psychopathology. This point is summarised well here by Sakheim and Devine (1995):

> A bioreductionist focus on the individual deflects attention away from social problems such as rape, war, child abuse, wife battering and violent crime. This leads to a channeling of resources toward understanding the 'pathology' of the victim rather than focusing attention on those who perpetrate abuse or on exploring the 'pathology' present in social systems that allow such abuses to occur . . . We do not label violence, war, sexism and persecution as 'crazy', only those who get injured by them. (Sakheim and Devine 1995: 255–6).

As Sakheim and Devine note, the individualisation of social pathology, which Wilkinson's work strives to reverse, is intrinsic to biomedical psychiatric knowledge. Below, we offer a corrective to this by examining the relationship between differential victimisation and mental ill-health under sections related to warfare, childhood abuse, adult–adult violence and hate crimes. All of these point to unequal life chances in relation to the loss of personal security and the experience of positive well-being. The evidence we review points up the multiple ways in which social divisions and unequal power relationships are imposed and maintained by violence. One consequence of these dynamics of oppression is that the mental health of victims is affected.

Warfare and the military persecution of civilians

Both of the World Wars during the twentieth century were followed by health and welfare reforms. Policies improving the lot of those with mental health problems has also been associated with warfare. The events of the First World War were linked to a turning point in psychiatric knowledge and its legitimacy for the State. Pauper lunatics had preoccupied the attention of the latter for a century. Political concerns about military efficiency began to overtake this older focus on the threat madness posed to the moral order of civil society. After 1914, there was a recognition that war-strain led to emotional breakdown in ordinary people (Stone 1985). During the 'Great War', between 4 per cent and 7 per cent of volunteer combatants were deemed to be suffering from 'shellshock'. This was later called 'combat neurosis' and is now commonly known as 'post-traumatic stress disorder' or 'PTSD'.

The strong empirical evidence about the pathogenic impact of war-strain on combatants challenged a bioreductionist position in psychiatry. Until the First World War, the asylum doctors, as part of a eugenic legacy, had emphasised inherited vulnerability to mental abnormality. A eugenic cultural view, supported by, but not limited to, medicine, in Europe and North America considered that a 'tainted gene pool' accounted for all forms of madness, criminality, alcoholism, epilepsy, physical disability, prostitution and idiocy (Forsythe 1990; Marshall 1990). Because those breaking down in the trenches were 'England's finest blood' – officers and gentlemen and volunteer lower ranks – the eugenic view was both illogical and a form of near-treason. As Keane (1998) notes, it is now clear, after nearly a century of studying traumatised combatants, that psychologically stable personalities can develop both acute and chronic mental health problems after exposure to war-zone life.

A singular emphasis upon the traumatisation of combatants was overtaken during the twentieth century, as the norms of military activity switched increasingly to civilian targets. Examples of this, during the Second World War, included the mass bombing of non-military populations and the persecution of civilians by military personnel. Examples, in the latter regard, include the torture and massacre of unarmed civilians, the rape of women in occupied territory and the mass warehousing, starvation and selective execution of particular civilian groups in labour and extermination camps.

To these deliberate acts of military persecution can be added the trauma created by dislocation, when refugees are forced to leave their homes during wars within, or between, nations. Since the Second World War, such events have recurred in such diverse places as Turkey, Nigeria, Vietnam, Cambodia, the Balkans, Somalia, Sudan and Rwanda. The sustained military persecution of civilian populations and the episodic creation of refugees are now hallmarks of modern warfare and account for far more deaths and physical and psychological ill-health than old-style armed fighting between combatants.

As far as planned civilian persecution is concerned, modern warfare has increasingly been linked to 'conditions of maximum adversity' (Levav and Abrahamson 1984). The German Holocaust set the paradigm for other persecutory States to follow. This pattern of events included assaults, which were physical (beatings, torture and starvation), psychological (fear of death, insults to self-worth), psychosocial (disruption of family and social networks) and cultural-religious (anti-Semitism).

On 27 March, 1942, Goebbels made the following record in his diary, about the 'Final Solution' to exterminate European Jewry, prescribed by Hitler and enacted by his loyal followers in the SS and some sections of the German Army occupying Soviet territory:

> If we didn't act against them, the Jews would destroy us. No other government and no other regime, was able to solve this problem ... Thank God *the war offers us possibilities which would have been barred to us in peacetime*. These we must now use. (Cited in Sereny 1995: 350, emphasis added)

Thus, under conditions of warfare, prewar prejudices, discrimination and 'hate crimes' can be transformed into grand and (temporarily) legitimate political strategies. Although this transformation mainly features racial, tribal or ethnic persecution, the Nazi regime extended this to a range of other groups, including homosexuals, religious minorities and political opponents.

The latter emphasis was found in subsequent military junta regimes (for example, in Argentina, Greece and Chile), where political opponents were tortured, raped and murdered by military personnel. Whilst the extermination of physically and mentally devalued people was limited to the Nazi period, all of the other forms of military persecution have been replicated in whole or part in other regimes since 1945.

The scale of this civilian destruction and trauma at the hands of State-military personnel in less than a century is vast (Glover 1999). By 1918, 800,000 German civilians had been starved to death by the

British naval blockade of food supplies. The Allied 'carpet' bombing of Germany in the Second World War killed 593,000 civilians, of whom 40,000 died in a single firestorm one night in Hamburg.

By 1945, over six million Jews had been gassed by the Nazis in their four Polish extermination camps, or shot or hanged in occupied Soviet territory, along with hundreds of thousands of Gypsies, Slavs, Jehova's Witnesses, homosexuals and political opponents. Two-thirds of the victims of this industrialised slaying of unarmed civilians were women and children, with even the newborn not being spared. Inestimable millions of others died in labour camps from hunger and exhaustion in both Hitler's Germany and Stalin's Soviet Union.

By 1950, 340,000 Japanese residents had died as a result of the two nuclear bombs dropped on Hiroshima and Nagasaki five years earlier by the US air force. The US were soon to inflict mass bombing on Cambodia and twenty-five years later, in the Cambodian civil war, up to 40 per cent of the population (around three million people) were killed by Pol Pot and his ruthless army. In 1992, the Serb army, spurred on by a self-righteous nationalist fervour, set up 17 camps in which 20,000 Bosnian women and girls were raped. In the same year, 1.8 million Bosnians became refugees in the wake of Serbian 'ethnic cleansing'.

The toll cited above from the twentieth century is illustrative, not exhaustive. The sheer scale of the State's capacity to terrorise and victimise unarmed civilians in its own territory and beyond is gigantic compared to that of individuals (whether or not they are mentally disordered). Between 1945 and 1990 there were 150 wars leading to the deaths of 22 million people, with multiples of this number surviving but traumatised (Goldson 1993). The recurring traumatic context of mass death and violation in whole civilian populations forms a recurrent existential backdrop for any survivor. As well as suffering the emotional fallout of the events, traumatised survivors become parents and are disabled in the task. This leads to demonstrable raised levels of distress and dysfunction not only in the primary victims but also in a postwar, second generation (Solkoff 1992).

One impact upon psychiatric knowledge of this switch to civilian targets is that the original military notion of 'shellshock' became more and more relevant as a diagnosis of PTSD for non-combatants.

The origins of PTSD can be traced to civilian populations, especially in relation to 'the concentration camp syndrome', as much as to the original notion of 'shellshock'. The destruction and trauma of the episodic industrialised military persecution of unarmed civilians made the invention of PTSD an inevitability. It is now commonplace for the diagnosis of PTSD to be applied in relation to victims of natural and man-made disasters, road traffic or industrial accidents, violent crime and sexual trauma.

The focus by some mental health professionals on trauma and PTSD has been a matter of critical debate. It has been argued that the victim–trauma relationship implicit in the concept of PTSD is more elaborate and less victim-blaming than the diagnosis of, say, 'borderline personality disorder'. The latter diagnosis entered the lexicon of the Diagnostic and Statistical Manual from the psychoanalytical wing of the American Psychiatric Association (Kroll 1988). By contrast, PTSD is a diagnosis which focuses much less on personality and much more on situational features (of trauma). At the same time, some feminist critics argue that PTSD still medicalises women's problems and renders social relationships as individual (for the latter to 'work through' or 'recover' from). Becker (2000) suggests that a diagnosis of PTSD still separates the victim from the socio-political context of their trauma and retains a victim focus which diverts analytical attention from oppressive forces.

Whether PTSD is seen as a liberating or mystifying diagnosis, there is no doubt that it emerged from a social context in which the stressors associated with violence became salient for professionals. Warfare has been the most obvious and dramatic of these. As we will see later, the diagnosis of PTSD has retained a cultural salience for professionals because of the pervasiveness of other traumatic stressors in civil society during peacetime.

Another linkage to the development of psychiatric knowledge from conditions of war is that of 'institutional neurosis' (Barton 1958). Barton was a medical student present at the liberation of the Nazi concentration camps. He noticed the stereotypical pacing of inmates and their unwillingness to move from squalid insanitary conditions into cleaner huts prepared by the Allied forces. Later, similar inmate conduct was to be identified by him in the mental hospital. The symmetry between large mental hospitals and concentration camps was brought together conceptually in Goffman's notion of the 'total institution' (Goffman 1961). Between them,

Barton and Goffman established the now elaborate discourse of 'institutionalisation'.

War and psychiatric knowledge have thus been inextricably linked. The shellshock problem shifted professional attention from psychosis to neurosis, and biological authority was temporarily displaced by talking treatments. Dysfunctional inmate concentration camp behaviour invited comparisons with life in mental hospitals and fed one aspect of social psychiatric knowledge. These environmentalist linkages were not the whole picture, as warfare also stimulated and reinforced a biodeterminist form of psychiatric knowledge.

Eugenic psychiatry was part of a conservative political process of segregation, sterilisation or extermination of those deemed to be genetically inferior. This eugenic orthodoxy was commonplace in both Europe and North America before the 1930s. German biological psychiatrists only extended its logic to a natural conclusion. The twin methodology and 'tainted gene pool' assumptions of the psychiatric geneticists Rudin and Kallmann in Germany during the Nazi period have since been incorporated fully into biological research into psychosis over the last fifty years in both European and North American psychiatry (Marshall 1990). Rudin, along with others in the German Medical Association, advocated 'involuntary euthanasia' for those 'devoid of meaningful life'. The work of Kallmann and Rudin lives on, however, within mainstream psychiatric genetics, with non-Nazi researchers (such as Slater, Gottesman and Shields) forming a postwar bridge to recent psychiatric genetics.

The violation of children

During childhood, the experience of neglect and sexual and non-sexual assault renders people prone to raised levels of distress and dysfunction in later life. In the richest country in the world, the USA, three to five children die every day from abuse and neglect. In 1994 in that country, nearly three million children were reported to child protection agencies as alleged victims of parental maltreatment (Wurtele 1999).

This is an area in which extensive empirical evidence coexists with mythology. For example, a media-fuelled focus on 'stranger danger' has reinforced a public belief that paedophilia exists pre-dominantly or solely outside family boundaries. Another example is the common belief that incest is less traumatising than stranger assault.

The practice of mental health professionals has not always favoured demystification in this regard. For example, psychoanalysis suffered a major setback to its credibility when it was established that Freud switched from believing the accounts of childhood sexual abuse given by his patients to a position which emphasised fantasy (Masson 1988). The area of childhood abuse has thus been served poorly by psychiatric knowledge, probably because of the individualisation error emphasised earlier by Sakheim and Devine. This error is high-lighted here by Katz and Watkins (1998):

> Child sexual abuse is one of the most common forms of child victimisation in the USA. Until the 1980s, the sexual abuse of children was regarded as a relatively rare event that was often neglected or trivialised by mental health professionals as a construction of the victim's Oedipal fantasies. It is now recognised as a real and all-too-frequent occurrence – one that researchers believe affects about one out of four girls in the USA and one out of every ten boys. (Katz and Watkins 1998: 291–2)

Community survey estimates of unwanted sexual contact with adults before the age of 18 vary from 38 per cent (Russell 1983) to 59 per cent (Wyatt 1985). In Wyatt's survey, the rate went up to 62 per cent when sexual contact with peers was included. In a New Zea-land survey, Anderson *et al.* (1993) found that 32 per cent of their sample had suffered such an experience before the age of 16.

Another indication of childhood sexual victimisation comes from lifetime prevalence studies of rape using the retrospective accounts of adult victims. The National Violence Against Women (NVAW) survey in the USA, conducted between 1995 and 1996, found that 21.6 per cent of first rapes occurred when the victim was less than 12 years of age and 32.4 per cent of first rapes occurred when the victim was 12–17 years (Tjaden and Thoennes 1998). The gender ratio of victims of sexual assault in childhood has been estimated to be between 1.5 and 3 females to every one male (Katz and Watkins 1998). Boys are more likely than girls to be molested by strangers, with girls being much more likely than boys to be victims of intra-familial abuse.

The age, gender and relation of victim and perpetrator characteristics are variable and constructed, to some degree, by methodological and reporting considerations. The reporting of these abusers
by their victims is not the same in community and clinical samples
and male victimisation may be underreported. Those seeking help
are more likely to be distressed by their biological father abusing
them (because of its psychological significance in relation to trust,
attachment and affection) (Mennen 1993). By contrast, one-off
stranger abuse may lead to no clinical presentation but be reported
in a community sample. Although the great majority of perpetrators
are male, more reports of female molesters are occurring (up to
10 per cent). Female assault is more likely to occur in the family
and with pre-pubescent boys as victims (Rudin *et al.* 1995).

Finkelhor (1979) found that having a stepfather doubled the
probability of female victimisation, and Anderson *et al.* (1993) found
that stepfathers were ten times more likely to abuse than biological
fathers. About 20 per cent of sexual abuse of minors is committed by
males before the age of 18 (Vizard *et al.* 1995). In detained samples
of molesters, 50 per cent admitted using unnecessary force during
their assaults on children (Marshall 1990). This highlights (as with
adult rape) that violence and power are evident often in an apparent-
ently erotic act. Indeed, the contempt and depersonalisation
common in molesters makes the term 'paedophilia' intrinsically
problematic, given that affection or genuine liking and respect are
usually far from the scene.

Grandfather abuse is part of the incest picture. Abusive elders are
generally extending their younger proclivities, with granddaughters
typically being targeted after daughters have grown up (Margolin
1992). As Clark and Mezey (1997) note, paedophilia is one of the
few crimes which does not decline in probability with age, even
though there is a common cultural assumption of libidinal loss in
older men. They found that perpetrators of child sexual abuse were
spread evenly through the adult age span.

The mental health consequences of maltreatment in childhood
are both immediate and distal. The first effects are on the incidence
of childhood presentations with cognitive deficits for age, academic
underperformance, behavioural problems, phobias, enuresis, depression and general anxiety states. The relationships with abusive
care-givers are intrinsically dysfunctional. In addition, maltreated
children show interpersonal difficulties with peers, being more likely

to be asocial or aggressive. Sexually abused children may also become prematurely sexual and sexually aggressive to others.

The distal effects of maltreatment are multiple. There is an increased probability that survivors will present with a range of adult mental health problems (compared to non-abused peers). The highly variegated presentation of survivors has led Sakheim and Devine (1995) to conclude that they represent a set of 'trauma-related syndromes'. For example, survivors of childhood maltreatment are more likely than non-abused peers to present later with PTSD symptoms, parasuicidal behaviour, drug or alcohol abuse, self-harm and depression (Widom 1998). Diagnoses of antisocial personality disorder (especially in men) and borderline personality disorder (especially in women) are both correlated with childhood maltreatment.

Those sexually, not just emotionally or physically, abused may manifest this range *and* other problems. For example, there is an increased presentation of medical complaints in adult life (Katz and Watkins 1998). Also, a third of those sexually abused proceed to become abusers themselves. Many victims can only offer sub-optimal parenting, creating a 'cycle of abuse and neglect'. Estimates of the presence of childhood sexual abuse in the histories of adult presenters to mental health services vary from 30 per cent to 70 per cent (Briere and Runtz 1987).

Warring intimacy

As with childhood abuse, empirical evidence and mythology coexist about domestic violence. For example, violence is gendered but perpetrators are not only heterosexual men (a dominant part of the literature about domestic violence). Another similarity with the area of childhood abuse is that mental health professionals do not always demystify the role of violence in their own everyday practices.

Domestic violence is a complex area with much of the clinical and legal studies being of heterosexual male partner batterers and murderers (Aldarondo 1998). However, studies of homosexual relationships appear to show equal or *higher* rates of partner violence in gay and lesbian communities. Lie and Gentlewarrior (1991) surveyed a community sample of 1099 lesbians and found that 52 per cent reported being victims and 57 per cent perpetrators. Similarly, Kelly and Washafsky (1987) found that 62 per cent of gay men reported partner violence. This compares with reporting rates of 20–30 per cent of partner violence in heterosexual relationships. Currently, these descriptive studies give us little insight as to why violence plays a part in so many homosexual partnerships.

Much more empirical work has been carried out on female than on male victims. This female-focused literature tells us that battered women are four times more likely to present to mental health agencies with depression, parasuicide and psychosomatic complaints than non-battered women. Three national surveys in the USA conducted in 1975, 1985 and 1992 indicate that the rate of male to female violence is declining and the perpetrator gender ratio is equalising (Kaufman *et al.* 1994; Straus *et al.* 1988).

Some studies even show that in heterosexual relationships, women may equal men as perpetrators (Morse 1995; Straus 1993). However, the NVAC survey noted earlier (Tjaden and Thoennes 1998) found that the ratio of female to male victims in intimate partner violence in the mid-1990s was around 3:1, with 22.1 per cent of women and 7.4 per cent of men in the sample reporting victimisation by a partner during their adult life. A third of heterosexual partner homicide involves female perpetrators (Browne and Williams 1993). This suggests that if there is an equalising tendency in the gender characteristics of perpetrators, *extreme* violence (leading to death or serious injury) is still significantly more likely to involve female victims. If some of the evidence about domestic violence might imply an equalising effect across gender and sexuality, this is not the case in relation to sexual violence, which is overwhelmingly perpetrated by heterosexual men on both known and stranger victims.

Men predominate as both victims and perpetrators in non-sexual assaults in public. The NVAW survey found that 1.9 per cent of women and 3.4 per cent of men had been physically assaulted in the previous 12 months (Tjaden and Thoennes 1998). This survey also found significant racial differences, with American Indians being the largest group of victims (male and female, sexual and non-sexual).

The literature examining the relationship between adult–adult violence and mental health impact suggest three dominant presentations: PTSD, depression and panic attacks. Within this picture there are gender differences (Kessler *et al.* 1994). Women are 2–15 times more likely than male victims to be diagnosed with PTSD. Women also present with post-traumatic distress earlier. Men typically present after witnessing physical assault or being involved in combat. Women more typically present after sexual assault or domestic violence. Whereas the lifetime prevalence of a diagnosis of PTSD ranges from 7.8 per cent to 12.3 per cent in the general population, in victims of violence the post-assault rate for sexual violence is around 50 per cent and physical attack 40 per cent (Acierno *et al.* 1998).

Separating depression and anxiety symptoms from one another or from PTSD is largely a methodological artefact of diagnostic practices and research aims. However, some studies looking at depression in women have found a five-fold increase in incidence in the wake of physical violence (Kilpatrick, Edmunds and Seymour 1992). In relation to panic attacks, Falsetti *et al.* (1995) found that 94.4 per cent of women meeting DSM criteria for panic disorder had a history of physical attack.

A final general point to make about the psychological impact of domestic violence is that, especially in heterosexual relationships, children are common secondary victims. They suffer both physically and psychologically. Attempts on the part of some children to intervene in parental violence means that minors from violent families are three to nine times more likely than peers from non-violent families to experience serious physical injury (Straus *et al.* 1988). Moreover, a family norm of violence increases the probability that children will become perpetrators, both within, and without, their family of origin. They are also at increased risk of receiving a diagnosis of attention deficit disorder, suffering educational failure and exclusion and being victims or perpetrators of school bullying (Hall and Lynch 1998).

Violent bigotry

We noted that during periods of war, racial or ethnic violence might be elevated to a military strategy. During peacetime, bigotry may underpin many opportunistic, and some planned, assaults and homicides. This may be a function of antipathies about skin colour, ethnic background, religion or sexuality. All or any of these can be motives for violence. Some policy statements about 'hate crimes' add gender to the list (United States Congress 1992). This very inclusive list basically designates hatred of any individual outside the social category of the perpetrator as the likely motive for the attack. To complicate matters, the raised salience of violence may lead to raised levels of reactive or defensive violence in some oppressed groups. For example, African-American men are overrepresented in violent criminal populations.

Hate crimes are more likely than other violent crimes to be associated with multiple perpetrators, with two-thirds of them involving two or more attackers (Levin and McDevitt 1993). Also revictimisation is common. Barnes and Ephross (1994) found that 90 per cent of a sample of victims had experienced multiple attacks. Few of these crimes are driven by a systematic political ideology aimed at ridding the world of 'deserving' victims. The great bulk are carried out by bigoted young men or teenagers thrill-seeking outside their own neighbourhood or by older bigots attacking those perceived to be infringing their local territory (Levin and McDevitt 1995).

The raised incidence of psychiatric outcomes for victims are similar to the other violent crimes discussed earlier (PTSD, anxiety and depression). In addition, victims are more likely than others to be angry about the injustice and to feel despair about an attack on an aspect of their identity (say their skin colour or sexuality), which is immutable. This brings in a *group* dimension to the trauma, with peers of victims experiencing raised levels of anxiety about potential attacks. Others in a shared victim community are thus violated vicariously (Craig and Waldo 1996).

The experience and fear of hate crimes is one important dimension of raised levels of distress in minority communities but not the only one. It can be added to others within a multifactorial 'minority stress hypothesis'. The latter also includes such factors as internalised oppression from the dominant group, stigma and discrimination. For example, Meyer (1995) demonstrates how these factors combine to produce suicidal or depressive outcomes in homosexual men.

Taking stock of the victimisation evidence

The first part of this chapter has summarised the evidence about victimisation, social divisions and their associated mental health consequences. Apart from amassing and appraising evidence there is a particular analytical challenge about understanding why this body of knowledge captures the public imagination and mass media headlines much less than the material we address in the second part of the chapter below.

It is not that violence is not newsworthy – quite the reverse. However, the immediate, larger elements of the political drama of war or the lurid detail of particular murder scenes are more salient for journalists than the dispersed and long-term subjective impact on victims. The routine nature of violence (especially in North American 'peacetime' society) and during modern warfare means that it is normalised. Only unusual events *within* that norm tend to gain wide publicity. 'Atrocities' are newsworthy but to some extent they legitimise the normal horror of a style of war, which now typically prioritises civilian victims. Violence is also commodified in sport and film outlets. As a cultural product, violence is as likely to be consumed as a palliative or stimulant by boxing, wrestling and film fans, as it is to symbolise a form of modern alienation and be recognised as a common source of distress and dysfunction.

Another overall point in the face of the evidence we have summarised is that the micro-processes of sexual and domestic violence and stranger assaults lend themselves more readily to a moral discourse from policy makers. By contrast, the role of *politicians* in waging, or gaining from, war is more likely to be framed as political necessity or even heroism. A British example was the political advantage gained by Thatcher after the Falklands War in 1982. As we write, Milosevic has been brought to The Hague court to face charges of war crimes. His defence is that he acted to protect the Serbian nation – a sentiment shared by his protesting supporters back at home. Pinochet's murderous Chilean regime has still not been brought to account, etc.

Thus, although civil and international wars are a common backdrop to psychological trauma for combatants and civilians alike, individual acts of violence in civil society are much more likely to be subjected to a close negative evaluation. For example, in the USA, many murderers are executed or wait on 'death row'. By contrast, politicians responsible for the torture and deaths of thousands evade justice and retain their freedom and citizenship and may even be regarded by their supporters as national heroes.

Dangerousness in psychiatric patients: the problem of amalgam data and other methodological limitations

In recent times, dangerousness has become a dominant public image about mental illness and risk management, a recurring focus in mental health policy. Fear in those not yet mad, or never to become so, is entwined with the image of the homicidal madman. This fear has been actively reinforced by the distorting effect of media relish, politicians keen to maximise their votes and conservative interest groups, such as some of those dominated by relatives of psychiatric patients. The British government, since 1997, has emphasised dangerousness in its mental health policy and advocated more and more restrictive powers in its reforms of legislation and services (Rogers and Pilgrim 2001).

A prejudicial, rather than an evidence-based, view of a purported linkage between diagnosed mental illness and raised levels of violent action has been underpinned by specifiable interests. Popular stereotypes about irrationality are one factor. If children are socialised from an early age to associate irrationality with aggression, then this is retained as a powerful image in later life, as unpredictable threat is feared more than that which is readily anticipated. The relatives of patients may be motivated, in part, about ensuring adequate *care* in local services by emphasising fears about inadequate levels of *control*. This blurring of care and control is easily made by pointing to a purported link between dangerousness and psychiatric diagnosis.

Faced with the need to develop credible policies about social order, politicians readily identify psychiatric patients as a definable group. Psychiatric patients are relatively powerless and their episodic loss of reason makes it easy for politicians to pick on a group which lacks social credibility in the eyes of others. If we are to transcend the traps set by the interplay of these prejudicial interests, we need to step back and examine what the evidence base is about psychiatric patients and dangerousness.

Moreover, there is an important pre-empirical logical consideration which is not commonly addressed by the courts or the psychiatric profession when making judgements in particular cases about the relationship between mental disorder and violence. Bean (1986) notes that, logically, if a person is judged to be both violent and mentally disordered, three scenarios are possible. First, they may remain violent after they are no longer adjudged to be mentally disordered. Second, they may cease to be violent but may still be adjudged to be mentally disordered. Third, their mental disorder and violence fluctuate over time in a correlated way. Bean notes that generally the first two contingencies are not explored and the third one is simply assumed to apply in all cases *and* the correlation is assumed to be causal and unidirectional. He correctly points out, then, that a person's mental state and their proclivity for violence may functionally be quite separate. The aggregate implication of the summation of the three scenarios is that violence and mental state are likely to be in an orthogonal relationship. Moreover, correlations may not be causal. They may be spurious or they may co-vary because of a third variable. Later, we examine ecological differences as a third set of variables.

Another implication of this public and political preoccupation with an examination of psychiatric populations for evidence of violence is that it obscures risk in the opposite direction. Psychiatric patients are more likely than non-patients to die as a result of homicide.

Turning, then, to the empirical evidence about dangerousness, it is important to disaggregate aspects of complex data. If *all* those managed by psychiatric services are put together, it is true that a modest relationship exists between psychiatric patienthood and violence. However, within such populations, for a variety of historical reasons, those who are prone by character to violence (with a diagnosis of anti-social personality disorder, or ASP) and those who abuse alcohol or disinhibiting illicit drugs (such as amphetamines, cannabis and 'crack' cocaine) may be managed by psychiatric services and receive a psychiatric diagnosis. Services do not *only* contain those with just variant diagnoses of psychosis or neurosis. Despite this aggregation of diagnoses in services, the general public may see all patients as being simply mentally ill (and dangerous).

A further complication is that the very small association between a diagnosis of psychosis (schizophrenia or bi-polar affective disorder) and violence contains its own amalgam. Some psychotic patients with some specific symptoms are more prone to violence than a general population. At the same time, others with a diagnosis of psychosis are *less* likely to be violent than a general population but may be at increased risk of victimisation and self-harm. Indeed, any risk of violence linked to psychosis alone is so small that it is contested. Some studies demonstrate this small association whereas others suggest no link, or even that psychotic patients are *less* violent than the general population.

Thus, to develop a clear picture of the empirical evidence, this complex amalgam has to be unpicked. In particular, the following groups of psychiatric patients have to be separated:

1. Psychotic patients who do not abuse alcohol or other disinhibiting substances,
2. Those with a primary diagnosis of personality disorder who are not deemed to be mentally ill,
3. Substance abusers who are not deemed to be mentally ill,
4. Those patients in whom psychosis, personality disorder and/or substance abuse coexist. In traditional psychiatric terms, this is called the problem of 'co-morbidity' or 'dual diagnosis'.

In a large study which compared amalgam with disaggregated information about psychiatric patients and violence, the following picture emerged (Swanson *et al.* 1990). The authors found that those with a diagnosis of psychosis alone (with no substance misuse or other dual diagnosis) were three times more violent than those without a psychiatric diagnosis. However, even in this group there was a low base rate of violence (7 per cent, i.e., 93 per cent of patients are not violent). The rate of violence was similar for sub-categories of severe mental illness (schizophrenia, bi-polar affective disorder and major depression). Those with a diagnosis of alcoholism were twelve times more violent than those with no diagnosis. Those with a diagnosis of drug abuse were sixteen times more likely to be violent than those without a diagnosis. This study highlights a central problem about amalgam data – diagnoses of *mental disorder* subsume dysfunctional and sometimes dangerous individuals who are not deemed to be *mentally ill*.

One of the reasons that the evidence has varied over time to confirm or disconfirm popular prejudice in this area is that, methodologically, there has been an insufficient separation of the four groups in the above list. All four groups may be recorded for social administrative purposes as being 'psychiatric patients'. Even with such a lack of separation, the undifferentiated link between those with any psychiatric diagnosis and violence has been described as 'modest'. Compared to other variables (young age, male gender, history of violence), psychiatric diagnosis (with the exception of anti-social personality disorder) is a weak predictor of dangerousness.

In relation to group 1 above, where studies find either no relation-ship between mental illness and violence or a very weak relationship, a question is still begged – *if* a small association does exist between a diagnosis of psychosis and an increased risk of violence, *which patient characteristics might be implicated*? This question is important because any success in precisely identifying risk factors in psychotic patients may prevent a group of patients (say, those with a diagnosis of 'schizophrenia') being coercively controlled or discriminated against *en masse*. Specific factors may enable clinical staff to avoid the civil liberty implications of this problem of overgeneralisation.

When all four groups are aggregated, a second question is this: when violence occurs at the hands of psychiatric patients, *which social processes might be implicated*? This question is important because it expands the frame about dangerousness to include a wider open social system implicating many variables which include, but are not limited to, patient characteristics. Monahan and Steadman (1994) point out that the research on violence and mental disorder is prone to several methodological difficulties.[1]

If we look at the evidence about patient variables alone, the clear-est predictor is not a diagnosis of mental illness but one of antisocial personality disorder (ASP), or in current British legal terminology, 'psychopathic disorder'. This is because the diagnosis is derived tautologically from antisocial actions which usually entail some form of sexual or non-sexual violence. The diagnosis relies on these behavioural indices – without them it is not made.[2]

In Britain, a range of other patients with a diagnosis of personality disorder other than ASP may also be contained or managed by psy-chiatric services. For example, those suffering from Munchausen's syndrome and Munchausen's-by-proxy and those committing crim-inal acts when in a dissociative state (the rarely diagnosed 'multiple personality disorder') may not receive a diagnosis of ASP but may be found in mental health services, as might those with a diagnosis of paranoid personality disorder (Pilgrim 2001).

Turning to the issue of psychosis and violence, this implicates groups 1 and 4 above (a diagnosis of psychosis alone or dual diagno-sis). Early studies of post-discharged psychiatric patients suggested that they were *less* likely than the general population to be arrested for assaults (Rabkin 1979). What might be important about Rabkin's review (which was a longitudinal look at a series of studies since the 1920s) is that the period before 1965 showed this 'less than average' picture of violence. However, after 1965 a reversal of findings occurred. This could be accounted for by the increased incidence of substance abuse generally in the population, especially in low social class groups in socially disorganised localities. These are the very ecological characteristics of many discharged patients in recent times. Prior to 1965, most patients were institutionalised and the community context contained less substance abuse.

More recent studies indicate that psychiatric patients *are* more likely than the general population to be arrested for violent assaults – the median ratio since 1965 has been just over 3:1 (Link *et al.* 1992; Stueve and Link 1997). The largest recent study to examine post-discharge rates of violence was by Steadman *et al.* (1998), who found that the dual-diagnosis group was more violent than the general population *and* those who abused substances without a diagnosis of mental illness. The implication of this is that when the psychosis-alone group and the dual-diagnosis group are aggregated, there is a raised risk of violence from post-discharged patients as a whole population, with the latter group giving the former one a 'bad name'. The Steadman *et al.* study indicated that 27.5 per cent of this amalgam group committed at least one violent act within a year. It also indicated quite clearly that the co-presence of substance abuse and/or underlying hostile personality characteristics is the constellation of variables which best predicts violence in some psychotic patients. According to the Steadman *et al.* study, sub-stance abuse nearly doubles the probability of violence in psychotic patients and more than doubles it in those with a diagnosis of personality disorder.

It is important to note here that *contra* the Swanson *et al.* study, which indicated a slightly raised risk of violence from a 'psychosis alone' group, the Steadman *et al.* study found that this group was no more likely to be violent than non-patient neighbours. Thus, a diag-nosis of psychosis *per se* leads either to no increased risk in violence or a minor elevation in risk. The large majority of psychotic patients are not violent for a number of reasons. First, psychosis is often linked to social withdrawal and, thus, potential contact with victims is less than the general population norm. For this reason, it is not surprising that patients with 'negative symptoms' are generally less violent than those with 'positive symptoms', as the latter are more likely to engage actively with others (Soyka 2000).

Second, most psychotic patients do not abuse illicit drugs or alcohol, although this does imply that the dual diagnosis population is numerically insignificant. Prevalence studies of psychotic patients abusing alcohol or illicit drugs suggest rates of between 20 per cent and 30 per cent (Hambracht and Hafner 1996). Epidemiological studies indicate that there is a three to fourfold increase in the risk of alcohol or other substance misuse in those with a diagnosis of schizophrenia or bi-polar affective disorder (Regier *et al.* 1990). The only diagnosis which has a higher correlation with substance misuse is – noted again here for our emphasis – that of ASP.

Third, not all psychotic patients who abuse drugs or alcohol are violent. The issue here is elevated *group risk* in dual diagnosis. The figures quoted earlier from Link *et al.* (1992) and from Steadman *et al.* (1998) demonstrate a statistical association in the dual-diagnosis *group*; they do not suggest that a dual diagnosis in *all* individuals predicts violent action. Some psychotic patients in the dual-diagnosis group are not violent and thus contribute to the non-violent portion of a psychiatric population.

An important question about the co-presence of ASP or substance abuse is that of the confidence entailed in attributing violence directly to psychotic symptoms and the ambiguous cause-and-effect relationship between parts of a dual diagnosis. Given that ASP and substance abuse are predictors of violence alone, in a particular dual-diagnosis psychotic patient it is often impossible to disaggregate the predictor variables (Soyka 2000). Also some psychiatrists now view drugs and alcohol as aetiological factors in psychosis (i.e., they are not merely co-present).

A further complication is the blurred line between the symptoms of one group, personality disorder, and that of another – psychosis. For example, paranoid personality disorder entails characteristics of suspiciousness and hostility. A person with this diagnosis may have episodes of deluded conduct but remain dangerous, even when delusions are not present, for example when holding a grudge and stalking a victim. A final feature to consider in the dual-diagnosis group is the raised level of non-adherence with anti-psychotic medication. Such non-adherence is a predictor of violence (Bartels *et al.* 1991; Swartz *et al.* 1998).

There has been evidence to suggest that some specific symptoms of psychosis predict violence, such as command hallucinations (Junginger 1995). Although the presence of delusions in general does not predict violence, those which contain hostile content, especially entailing a fixed victim or victims, may be predictive (Taylor 1985). By contrast, Applebaum *et al.* (1999) did not find that delusions predicted violence but they did find that a 'suspicious' attitude towards others was a long-term predictor. This is not surprising because those who are not deluded but by temperament are suspicious may be both hostile and sufficiently rational to deliberate on victimising others. However, other studies have failed to confirm that specific psychotic symptoms predict violence (Teplin 1990).

The clinical literature suggests that, as with the general population, most perpetrators are male (Blumenthal and Lavender 2000; Silver *et al.* 1999). Muntaner *et al.* (1998) found in relation to all arrests (not just violence) that men were significantly overrepresented in inpatient populations who had drug-induced psychosis. However, some studies show slightly more female violence in discharged patients (Lidz *et al.* 1993) and even higher female rates in secure facilities (Larkin *et al.* 1988). Other studies of inpatients show no sex differences (Tardiff and Sweillam 1982) – see Stueve and Link (1998) for an account and interpretation of these mixed findings.

An interpretive difficulty with studies of inpatient regimes is the wide range of findings across time and place. For example, in Britain risky behaviour (especially the dual-diagnosis group pointed up by Muntaner *et al.* (1998)) has increasingly characterised acute units in the past ten years with competition for limited bed space (Rogers and Pilgrim 2001). However, recent Italian findings show low rates of inpatient assaults (only 6 per cent prevalence) (Raja *et al.* 1997). Most of the research on violence in open settings has been undertaken in the USA.

Spector (2001) reviewed the literature about attitude to race and violence when staff assess psychiatric patients and found that they show some bias in this regard. In particular, young Afro-Caribbean males are judged to be more dangerous than whites with similar symptom profiles. Thus, not only do violent outcomes seem to vary in the findings about mental health facilities but there are also biases in the prediction of violence within these settings.

To conclude this section on clinical variables: a diagnosis of psychosis *per se* in a patient signifies only a small elevation of raised risk of violence compared to a substantial elevation in ASP and substance abuse patients (and some non-psychiatric sub-groups of the general population). However, there is some evidence that some specific symptoms may be risk predictors but even this is contested (for example, conflicting findings on delusions). Compliance with medication is certainly a risk predictor. Diagnoses of ASP and substance abuse disorder are much better predictors of violence than those of schizophrenia or bi-polar affective disorder alone. The association between psychiatric diagnosis and violence becomes very strong in those with 'co-morbidity'.

This section also begs a question: if there is a slightly raised risk of violence in psychotic patients in the community, might the latter be making a substantial ecological influence (which we might wrongly attribute to clinical variables alone)? We now turn to this ecological question.

Patient variables, dangerousness and the wider social context

Bearing in mind the methodological limitation noted earlier about constricted validation samples (patients are studied more often than other social groups), some studying violence in the mental health field have argued for an extended or elaborated systemic framework. This expands our frame of reference beyond patient variables and explores pathways to violence in an open social context (a point we cited from Wilkinson (2000) at the start of the chapter). Silver *et al.* (1999) considered the issue of patient dangerousness in the light of the literature on locality differences in the base rate of violence. The latter suggests that poor, socially disorganised neighbourhoods not only have higher levels of crime but also develop a stronger cultural norm of violence. The latter 'code of the streets' may be seen as a normal means to resolve conflicts, as well as a vehicle for some types of acquisitive crime such as mugging and aggravated burglary. Psychiatric patients are more likely to be found in such poor localities because they are often permanently excluded from the labour market. Consequently, like other residents in these areas, they are at a higher risk (compared to those in more stable and affluent neighbourhoods) of being both the victims and perpetrators of violent crime.

Silver *etal.* (*ibid.*) followed up 293 discharged patients in Pittsburgh and found that certain *individual* variables were associated with raised levels of violence. Men were more violent than women. African-Americans were identified as being more violent than whites. Those with previous arrests for serious crimes were more likely to be violent. Those who abused alcohol or street drugs or who had a diagnosis of ASP were significantly more violent.

When they looked at ecological variables, they found that overall those discharged to poorer areas were more than twice as likely to be violent as those to non-poor areas. Moreover, some of the individual predictors, such as race, disappeared in interaction with the ecological picture. In richer areas, African-American patients were no more violent than white patients. However, some of the individual and ecological variables interacted positively. Those patients with drug or alcohol problems, prior arrests and a diagnosis of ASP were significantly more likely to be violent in poor areas than in richer areas. Unlike other studies, the Silver *etal.* cohort did not demonstrate effects for age and socio-economic status.

This study highlights the importance of understanding violence (like any other form of behaviour) in its social context. It may be that the professional and political focus of attention on clinical variables alone creates analytical blinkers about a complex open system which involves many ecological variables operating separately and together in interaction with patient variables. For example, if the normative structure of a locality is one of violence, patients will be influenced by this potentially as both perpetrators and victims.

The work of Virginia Hiday exemplifies this open-systems approach (Hiday, 1995). Figure 6.1. above is offered by Hiday as a broad framework of understanding. Hiday's model involves what she calls 'violence-inducing social forces' (*ibid.*: 127). These forces not only shape psychotic symptoms (triggers for relapse), they also shape non-psychotic action, such as violence. The latter shaping process is as true of non-patients as patients who reside in areas which Silver *etal.* (1999) describe as being characterised by 'concentrated poverty'.

Hiday also notes that poverty is not merely about one moment of material deprivation captured by, say, a social survey of socio-economic status. It also signifies a chronic cumulative process of subjective disaffection with life. The latter entails a common experience in (all) poor people of anomie and a lack of personal control.

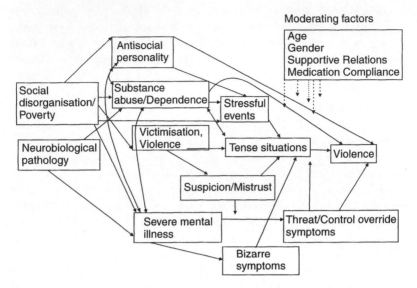

Figure 6.1   Causal model linking social stratification with mental illness and violence
Source: Hiday 1995. Reproduced with permission.

These subjective experiences are then compounded by a lack of social opportunities to leave poverty by legal means, as well as the direct impact of financial poverty. These direct economic variables increase the probability of all forms of ill health and mediate the negative health impact of poor diet and the comforts of drugs and alcohol. Thus, poverty has a double effect – one related to external stressors which affect well-being and another to do with the hopelessness and fatalism created by chronic deprivation (see Chapter 5).

The review and model of Hiday also reinforce a point we made earlier, that substance abuse or alcohol abuse are predictors of violence. If these features are then medicalised, as DSM-defined disorders managed by a medical speciality (psychiatry), they will be recorded as *psychiatric* variables which predict violence. This blurs the distinction in the public's mind about one group of patients who have a high probability of violence and another group of patients that does not. This is not merely a matter of public prejudice, as the social organisation of mental health services to date in North America, Europe and Australasia has been about the former patient group and not just those with a diagnosis of psychosis. This returns us to the problem of amalgam data associated with the broad concept of 'mental disorder'.

A final point to emphasise about the context of violence is the data on the *victims* of patient violence. Whilst the spectre of stranger attacks by mad people may drive a vote seducing mission, when some politicians construct mental health policy and may dominate the anxious mentality of the general public, the empirical reality is that, as with non-psychiatric populations, intimacy is the key to prediction (Estroff and Zimmer 1994). Moreover, within this empirical reality, patients are much *less* likely to attack strangers than are non-patient perpetrators. When psychiatric patients do commit violent acts, most victims are already known to them, with estimates varying from 80 per cent (Gottlieb *et al.* 1987) to 95 per cent (Lindqvist and Allebeck 1990). In the latter study, it was found that non-psychiatric attackers were *five* times more likely to target a victim not known to them than patient perpetrators.

Differential population disadvantage

The discussion above about the reversal of post-1965 findings on the link between mental disorder and violence highlighted two issues. The first relates to raised levels of substance and alcohol abuse in the general population, which is reflected in and impacts upon psychiatric patients. The second is the living circumstances of discharged patients. With deinstitutionalisation, many psychiatric patients, because of their disadvantaged labour market position, have been resettled or begun to live in the community in a non-random way. That is, they are more likely to be accommodated in poor localities (see Chapter 2).

This poor locality picture has implications. As the Hiday model above indicates, it brings psychiatric populations into disproportionate contact with factors which increase risk in *both* directions. Inevitably, they are more likely to be *victims* of crime in high crime areas and they are more likely to encounter perpetrator risk predictors, especially illicit drugs.

Several studies have demonstrated that clinical populations in the community are at a higher risk of violent victimisation than the general population, most of which is accounted for by differential ecological effects (Hiday *et al.* 2001). In the other direction, those patients with a diagnosis of ASP, as well as other violent offenders without the diagnosis, are disproportionately settled in poorer areas. The controversy in Britain in the summer of 2000 about paedophiles on poor council estates highlighted this point. The resettlement of violent offenders in poorer areas increases the risk to all people in a locality (including psychiatric patients residing there with no violent history).

Thus, risk is socially structured by place as well as actor variables, and these interact. The base rate for violence varies from place to place. Urban areas are more violent than rural areas. Within cities, some parts are more violent than others. The demographic features of actors that predict violence (male gender, young age, race, unemployment, low socio-economic status and poor education) are differentially structured by locality.

For example, young unemployed, poorly educated males are more likely to be on the streets of poor areas than richer localities. Variations occur in the public presence of risky actors, so that in conditions of darkness such groups are also more likely to be intoxicated or under the influence of illicit drugs. Monahan (1993) has described the interrelationship between such commonly coexisting variables in violent actors as a 'ball of wax' problem – it is difficult to disentangle particular predictors, and cause and effect become entwined.

A young man who is poor is more likely to be poorly educated and be chronically unemployed. He is more likely to live in an area with high substance abuse. His unemployed anomie gives him both time to enact crime and a lack of consideration about its impact on his fellow citizens. His violent crime may be motivated by some combination of thrill-seeking, material gain or the need to feed a drug habit. His drug habit leads to disinhibition making violence easier, etc.

Violence and coercion

A final way in which psychiatric patients may suffer differential life chances about violence is in relation to the State's decision-making affecting them as perpetrators. Not only is mental health policy often skewed more towards control than care in its funding priorities, the legal framework for dealing with mentally disordered offenders is discriminatory. For example, mentally disordered offenders lose their liberty for at least as long as an imprisoned perpetrator of a similar offence and often more. The detention of mentally disordered offenders is open-ended, whereas for those going to a prison, 'disposal' sentences are fixed and prescribed. The rules governing lawful interventions in prisons and hospitals are different. Forced medication in response to disruptive conduct may be seen as an assault in a prison but considered a therapeutic intervention in a hospital.

Another differential effect is in relation to the 'ball of wax problem' noted by Monahan (1993). If it is difficult to isolate risk factors that can be targeted by the State's social control policies in high-crime areas, it is *not* difficult to identify people with a psychiatric diagnosis. For example, we have dedicated mental health law to remove people from society without trial (whether or not they have committed an offence). We do not have laws to remove the liberty, without trial, of poorly educated unemployed young men, with no psychiatric diagnosis, who drink excessively in the evening. This group contributes substantially more to violence in society than do psychiatric patients. If all members of this group of young men were obliged to take major tranquillisers, their rate of offending would probably decrease.

Thus, whilst the amalgam data on mental state is only a 'modest' predictor of violence (and that on psychosis alone poor), it is a very good predictor of the occurrence of selective social control. Recently, the British government has been proposing a curfew system to reduce the antisocial actions of young people. This has produced a substantial controversy as a civil liberty issue. By contrast, 'therapeutic law' is taken for granted as part of the State's legislative apparatus in most countries.

Suicide

In the final section of this chapter, we address the issue of homicidal violence against the self. Suicide has a particular salience in debates about mental health and inequalities for two reasons. First, it is sometimes the main or singular governmental population measure of mental health. In 1998, suicide reduction was set as a World Health Organization priority (WHO 1998). In Britain during the 1990s, both Conservative and Labour governments set suicide reduction targets as the main societal level goal of mental health improvement (DoH 1999).

Second, there has been considerable debate about the ambiguous relationship between individual psychopathology and the social conditions associated with attempted and completed suicides. Those with a diagnosis of severe mental illness have a raised probability of suicide. It is not clear, though, whether this reflects the social alienation and poverty of psychiatric patients or that suicide is mainly a function of the irrational decision making of those who are mentally ill (or both).

If suicide is only debated as a social policy question in terms of assumed irrationality (a proxy for mental illness), then this is overly restrictive and does not do conceptual justice to its complexity. Moreover, such a narrow conflation of suicide with mental illness or psychopathology is not supported by the empirical evidence. Most completed suicides are *not* by those with a recent diagnosis of mental illness, although there is a strong correlation with past mental health service contact.

Outside the social policy and psychiatric discourse, we find those who argue for suicide as a *non-pathological* social phenomenon. Camus raised the matter of the choice over one's life or death to a high philosophical plain. Durkheim argued for a range of types of suicide which became more or less prevalent according to societal conditions. According to Durkheim, suicide might reflect altruism in a highly regulated society (such as *hara-kiri* in Japan) or anomie in those socially excluded in conditions of poor social integration.

Estimates of suicide risk, based on clinical and actuarial variables combined, have not been very successful to date. For example, O'Connor *et al.* (1999) examined 142 completed suicides and found that only 15 per cent complied with the expectations of clinically depressed older males with a psychiatric history. Similarly, Pokorny (1983, 1993) traced the survivability of 4800 patients over a five-year period and, using the best risk assessment means available from psychiatric epidemiology, could only make predictions about *individual patients* at a slightly better level than chance.

This is not to say that psychiatric populations are not more prone to suicide. There is a 14-fold increase in the risk of suicide for those with a diagnosis of schizophrenia (for both sexes), and for those with a diagnosis of a major affective disorder there is a 12-fold increase for men and 16-fold for women (Baxter and Appleby 1999). However, suicide occurs in many non-psychiatric populations as well. Moreover, it is a low probability event in both populations. Therefore, purely on logical grounds, suicide should not be a naive proxy measure for mental health or mental illness.

Whilst its conceptual status (a social or psychiatric phenomenon?) and its genesis might be a focus of controversy, suicide is undoubtedly a form of violence. As with violence to others, we find that it is not only partially predicted by mental state but is also predicted by non-psychiatric variables, such as poverty, age, gender and employment status. However, it should be emphasised that suicide is more strongly associated with a diagnosis of mental illness than is violence to others.

As with the Hiday diagram on violence (see Fig. 6.1), it is possible to situate mental state within an open system of other variables which interact to increase the chances of suicide (a 'synergy' effect). However, most of the time these variables interact to produce a non-suicide outcome. Suicide, even in high risk groups, is a low probability behaviour. Although there has been a steady rise in suicide rates in developed countries over the past few decades, only around 10 people per 100,000 kill themselves each year (O'Connor and Sheehy 2001). Most psychiatric patients, just like most recently unemployed people, do not commit suicide, even though both groups are at a greater risk.

Approaches within clinical psychology have offered some bridging concepts between psychiatry and sociology. Psychiatrists who point out the raised prevalence of suicide in those with a diagnosis of depression or schizophrenia cannot account for why most with these diagnoses do not end their own lives. Similarly, those only emphasising variants of social stress, intrinsic to Durkheimian arguments, cannot account for why most people in such high risk social contexts still do not kill themselves.

One response to such ambiguity is for psychoanalytical writers to explore the particular self-destructive psychodynamics of those who die by their own hand (Firestone 1997). More cognitively oriented psychologists suggest mediating variables related to a cognitive style in suicidal people of hopelessness. This style is associated with a tendency to generate negative predictions about the future and an impeded capacity to generate positive predictions.

This hopelessness bias in decision making seems to be present in suicidal individuals independent of a diagnosis of depression. Apart from feeling hopeless about the future, suicidal individuals are also more likely to have a poor self-image and to blame themselves for difficulties in their lives. This combination of hopelessness and self-blame leads to suicidal people being inefficient at problem solving about the difficulties in their social situation. Also, their autobiographical accounts raise the salience of general negative views of their personal history and lower the probability of recall of specific events, which might be positive and introduce complexity to the general memory and be a building block for positive future scenarios (Williams 1997).

A final cognitive feature of those who seem to be more at risk of suicide is that of 'socially prescribed perfectionism' (Dean and Range 1999). Those who are too perfectionist will never be satisfied with the standards set for them. Consequently, positive future scenarios would disconfirm their identity and tend to be discarded in favour of safer negative ones. What is currently not clear, empirically, is the relative salience of social learning and biological susceptibility in individuals with these cognitive biases.

These psychological accounts of suicidal people have mainly focused on the large overlap between depressive ways of thinking (combined with perfectionism) leading to suicidal ideation which might proceed to suicidal action. Less has been investigated about those with a diagnosis of schizophrenia. In the latter group, their self-absorption may combine with social exclusion to generate a hopeless scenario. What both groups have in common is access to psychiatric drugs which can be used in lethal overdose (though latterly, anti-depressant drugs which are less toxic than early versions are more often prescribed).

Those who use illicit drugs alongside prescribed medication are vulnerable to accidental death from their interaction. For this reason, there are administrative problems about the accurate recording of cause of death when people die from drug over-doses.

Monahan's 'ball of wax' metaphor about violence to others applies also to suicide within open systems. For example, a person who has suffered abuse in childhood may become depressed and as a result fail to hold down a job. Their chronic unemployment makes them impoverished materially and weakens their social networks. Their earlier abuse leads them to dwell on a general sense of disappointment about the past. Their restricted, depressive style of thinking makes everyday problem-solving arduous. A sense of growing incompetence in the latter regard confirms the negative view the person already has of himself or herself. The person seeks short-term comfort in the solitary drinking of alcohol. The latter depresses mood and creates recurring toxic reactions. This overall set of factors combines to produce a hopeless scenario. The hopelessness is partly objective and partly subjective as well as being partly physical, partly psychological and partly social.

In the above small vignette we can see objective events, past and present, becoming combined with inner events for a person who is subjected to but also participates in social processes. Suicide is an event much like turning into a blind alley and fatally crashing a car into a dead-end wall. What has shaped this event can be traced to both the restricted roads available to them (objective conditions past and present in their lives) and the driver's limited map reading (their cognitive style prone to negative scenario building). The roads which have shaped the fateful route include all of the features we know predict low self-esteem and restricted options (actual and perceived). These features might include labour market fluctuation as well as the quality of parenting, early bereavement, abuse and neglect in childhood, current employment status, masculine identity, current life events, etc.

Thus, a constant interplay between social conditions and personal experience makes events such as suicide and biographical experiences such as depression impossible to disentangle from an external set of factors that shape and constrain action (Pilgrim and Bentall 1999). They are part of the ball of wax noted already. The multifactorial model of violence from Hiday is similar to that offered by Brown and his colleagues when studying depression in working-class women. For Brown *et al.* (1995) a defining end-point feature (for them clinical depression) is that of entrapment. That is, the depressed person feels that they cannot leave a field of oppressive conditions. Suicide is an irrevocable way of leaving the field when there appears to be no other way out.

The above account of suicide then suggests the following:

- Suicide is not necessarily, or even usually, a symptom of recent mental illness but those with a psychiatric history are at greater risk than those without,
- The social variables which predict suicide are similar, but not identical, to those implicated in violence to others,
- Suicide is a discrete event but its antecedent conditions need to be conceptualised as social and psychological processes or continua which are also implicated in non-suicidal outcomes,

- The 'successful' suicide brings closure into an untenable, hopeless scenario. The latter is partly created by forces outside the individual and partly created by their cognitive style or a biographical trajectory of self-destruction,
- Suicide is one, but not the only, response to the experience of entrapment,
- Theories of suicide are vulnerable to psychiatric, psychological and sociological reductionism. Just as the suicidal individual brings *practical* closure into a complex open system, individual academic disciplines can bring *epistemological* closure into this complexity in their accounts of suicide.

Conclusion

This chapter set out to rebalance the discussion created by politicians, the mass media and some interest groups about mental disorder and violence. It explored victimhood and its relationship to distress and dysfunction. It tested a collusive prejudicial view against the evidence to date about psychiatric patients as perpetrators of violence. The first part of the chapter also highlighted that unequal power relationships are often characterised by violence: the armed State against the unarmed citizen; adults against children; intimate partners against one another; men against women and children; bigots against their hated targets.

Whilst these political fracture lines in society are important, politicians in particular have much to gain from maintaining a biased discussion by minimising the first on the list and raising the salience of the social problems linked to the others. In relation to victimhood, they can selectively focus on features in a governed population (such as domestic violence) but evade the mental health implications of their own decision-making in relation to warfare. They can also selectively attend to powerless parts of the population, such as psychiatric patients, and overvalue the contribution this group makes to violence in society.

The political emphasis on suicide has brought with it another distortion in which individual pathology is overemphasised. As a population level indicator of mental health, suicide is crude and inappropriate. However, its dramatic simplicity as a measure (dead or alive) and its emotive content about risk management seem to have encouraged its over-use by politicians. Indeed, risk management of an identifiable group (those with a psychiatric diagnosis), rather than the reduction of distress or the production of mental health gain, seems to have been the dominant feature of mental health policy both before and after deinstitutionalisation.

7

Professional and lay knowledge

Introduction

This chapter will explore the relationship between the knowledge-base of the mental health professions and aspects of inequality. Our book is mainly concerned with inequality in its traditional sense about disadvantage, exclusion and social oppression. However, within the domain of professional practice there is another set of related questions about power differentials and the ways in which forms of professionally preferred knowledge warrant some accounts about social inequality and discount others. The recent rise of lay or user knowledge in which the experience of individuals is privileged presents a challenge to the more professionalised bodies of knowledge underpinning the disciplines of mental health.

The chapter allows us some opportunity to identify ways in which inequality is embedded in the normal activity of professionals in their dealings with their client group. Because the medical speciality of psychiatry has dominated the mental health industry, we will focus on its knowledge-base in the main. Later in the chapter, we will also consider the ways in which other mental health professionals understand their work. We will examine the tension between the two dominant epistemological roots within psychiatric thinking (eugenics and psychoanalysis) and consider the success of the compromise of the biopsychosocial model. Finally, we explore briefly the way in which lay knowledge about mental health provides a focus both similar to and different from that of mental health professional knowledge.

Tensions and compromise in psychiatric expertise

In 1977, an influential book, *Psychiatry in Dissent*, ended a contentious decade within and about the psychiatric profession. Its author, the urbane Irish academic psychiatrist Anthony Clare, went on to become probably the best known mental health broadcaster in mainland Britain. Clare's work has a double significance as a case study. First, it has led to the assumption on the part of lay people that all psychiatrists are universal experts in *any* aspect of the mind and that they are all sophisticated in therapeutic conversations. This image was manifest in both of Clare's best known contributions on BBC's Radio Four: *All in the Mind* and *In the Psychiatrist's Chair*. It is hardly surprising that one source of disappointment in people with mental health problems hearing such programmes is that what they typically encounter in actual services are cursory administrative interviews and medication reviews. Clare's work, along with Hollywood stereotypes of psychiatrists being psychoanalysts, inadvertently may have led the average new psychiatric patient up the garden path.

Second, Clare's book produced a British compromise about 'anti-psychiatry'. Being neither in favour of the reductionist biodeterminism within psychiatric orthodoxy nor supportive of the wilder excesses of politicised psychoanalysts within his profession, such as Ronald Laing, Clare instead offered a 'portmanteau model' (Baruch and Treacher 1978). This can be contrasted with the angry defence of psychiatric orthodoxy against the threat of anti-psychiatry evident in contemporary responses from other professional leaders (e.g., Hamilton 1973; Roth 1973). The eclectic portmanteau model went on to gain respectability, particularly amongst social psychiatrists and in centres of excellence of psychiatric training – the integration of biological, psychological and social reasoning about mental illness.

This integrationist approach had been advocated in a less populist way several years previously by Adolph Meyer (and his 'psycho-biology'). Meyer influenced key psychiatric teachers in Britain before and after the Second World War, especially Henderson and Gillespie (in Scotland) and Lewis, one of Clare's teachers at the Institute of Psychiatry. (Lewis is cited in *Psychiatry in Dissent* but not Meyer himself.) This Meyerian influence reappeared subsequently in texts written not only by eclectic psychiatrists such as Clare but also by social workers and psychologists collaborating with them

(Falloon and Fadden 1993; Goldberg and Huxley 1980). It was also formalised by Engel (1980) as a means of reconciling science and humanism by creating a new model, which was holistic. This suggests that the biopsychosocial model has created some credible bridge building with some competing mental health professions and has also been an attempt to rescue psychiatry from the excesses of biological reductionism. The 'biopsychosocial model' does not discount madness-as-illness (a rejection popularised by the psychiatrist and psychoanalyst Thomas Szasz (1961)), nor does it remove the professional mandate of medicine to diagnose and authoritatively manage patients. What it reflects is an attempt on the part of one part of the leadership of the psychiatric profession to avoid the implosion of its knowledge-base made weak by the offence created by biological reductionism, whilst retaining a unified medical authority.

The tension between a biomedical approach and ones emphasising psychological or social explanations of mental health problems began to dog the psychiatric profession after the First World War, when the 'shellshock' problem had thrown the eugenic Victorian legacy into confusion (Stone 1985). On the one side were those still convinced that mental illness was a brain disease, assuredly caused by inherited defects, which warranted unfettered medical paternalism. On the other side were those who saw mental illness as being socially derived from current stressors and/or from interpersonal difficulties in the incipient patient's family. This led, in Anglo-American psychiatry, to recurring disputes between biological psychiatrists, medical psychotherapists and social psychiatrists. Within the American Psychiatric Association, biomedical champions have toughed it out with psychoanalysts for the last fifty years.

If the reader were to enter a library and peruse the contents of specialist biomedical psychiatric texts and then psychoanalytical books and journals, they would be struck by the self-confident detail in both genres. Both, in their own way, presume that reality has already been proven, whether this is about pathological brain functioning or psychosexual fixation and regression. Both are expressing certainty about what actually remains uncertain – the nature of madness and misery and their origins in *particular individuals*. While these bids for pre-eminence in the psychiatric profession lead to premature forms of arrogant knowledge claims in books and journals, the underlying uncertainty has practical consequences, as was noted here by Bassuk and Gerson (1978), writing at the time of *Psychiatry in Dissent*:

> The very nature of many conditions psychiatrists attempt to treat is still not well understood. In view of this lack of basic knowledge, it is not surprising that there are no accepted guidelines for establishing comprehensive systems for the delivery of mental healthcare – notably systems for reaching disadvantaged people (Bassuk and Geerson 1978: 47).

This quotation was cited by Light (1985) in his review of the tensions within American psychiatry about its training. In the US context, Light traced an enthusiasm for psychosocial ideas in the 1960s followed by a reactive 'return to medicine', which has continued until today.

The return to medicine after the 1960s

A number of commentators within the profession had lamented the unhelpful tensions and fragmentation created by sociological, psychotherapeutic and biomedical debates during the 1960s (Braceland 1977; Grinker 1975). What followed about this uncertainty and its potentially damaging internecine disputes, apart from progressive writers such as Clare advocating the biopsychosocial approach, was a 'return to medicine'. Fernando (1992), a writer on race and psychiatry, reflecting on his profession being attacked from many sides over a twenty-year period, argued that it had defensively:

> turned in on itself, going back to the traditional basics of medicine-emphasising biological and genetic aspects of health and illness, concentrating on drug therapy (as an undeniably 'medical' form of treatment) devising more and more specialisms and refusing to address serious problems (such as racism) within its professional practices. (Fernando 1992: 14)

In Chapter 8, we return to the question of how a variety of interests coincide to maintain a biomedical orthodoxy in psychiatry. The question begged is why does the biopsychosocial approach retain such a legitimacy in the writings of 'progressive' academic psychiatrists if the main camps in the profession still remain divided by the old tensions noted by Grinker and Braceman? The answer must reside in its functional advantages for professional rhetoric and disciplinary solidarity: it allows biological, psychological and social determinism to coexist and creates the outward appearance of wholism and evenhandedness about aetiology and treatment. But, as we noted above, detailed and certain aetiological accounts, even eclectic ones, of individual distress or madness are suspect or contestable.

The elusive nature of madness and misery and shifting cultural meanings attributed to their definition and genesis render professional knowledge claims provisional, contestable and bounded by time and space (Kleinman 1988). The gap between psychiatry's aspiration to be a respected medical speciality incrementally generating more valid knowledge-claims in its area of claimed expertise and its actual credibility amongst medical colleagues and mental health services users poses a problem for the profession. In recent years, orthodox psychiatric theory and practice have been attacked: by internal dissenters (the 'anti-psychiatrists' in Britain, the US, France and Italy); by competing professions (especially clinical psychology); and by a new social movement of disaffected service users. Psychiatrists as a professional group are the least popular of all professional groups in the eyes of people with mental health problems and are described as the least helpful of all parties – other patients are described as more helpful (Rogers *et al.* 1993).

The summary made by Fernando above is reminiscent of a similar point made by Light (1985) about psychiatric training in the 1970s in the US, indicating that there had been a 'return to medicine'. Light cites the statement made by the American Psychiatric Association in 1975 about training, which indicates that for a while psychoanalytical and not biomedical ideas were dominant:

> the psychiatrist is characterised by the medical assets he [*sic*] brings to the treatment of his [*sic*] patients. His distinct training includes patient responsibility, knowledge of psychodynamics, a cultivated sense of human growth and development, a heightened awareness of interpersonal process, professional objectivity, expert interviewing techniques and experience in negotiating counter-transference phenomena (American Psychiatric Association 1975; cited in Light 1985).

As Light points out, this list of vague and empirically unproven positive traits ('medical assets') is not even inherently medical, as psychological therapists from a variety of disciplinary backgrounds might make a similar claim. Indeed, critics of the brutalising effects of medical training might argue that it is antithetical to the development of the list of benign attributes being claimed. The list is also a good exemplar of a conservative 'trait' approach within the sociology of the professions in which a profession is depicted as being nothing but the public relations account it wants to give of itself at a particular time (Saks 1983).

Professional knowledge and inequalities

The above sections have introduced the problematic nature of psychiatric knowledge. This section examines the implications this has for inequality under the following sub-headings:

* the power imbalance created by professional knowledge
* psychiatric knowledge, medical dominance and individualisation
* normative knowledge and social control
* knowledge and status differentials in the mental health professions.

The power imbalance created by professional knowledge

Although knowledge about mental health is contested, the biological psychiatrist and the psychotherapist have in common their power over the patients they see. This micro-political asymmetry is common to all professionalised healers in relation to their client group and is not peculiar to the field of mental health. However, there are a couple of special features within this common picture.

First, because attributions about mental ill health are about the total self (not one fragment, as in having a broken leg), diagnosis and treatment have a particular totalising salience. This is why receiving a psychiatric label is peculiarly stigmatising – to be formally declared to have lost one's reason ensures that one's social credibility is permanently affected or, in some cases, lost completely (Ingleby 1981). Because of what is at stake, there have been sensitivities about psychiatric labelling. For example, much of the debate about mental health legislation at the turn of the twentieth century revolved around unfair detention of the sane. After that, public concern and professional unease focused upon psychiatric diagnosis and treatment being applied inappropriately to other cases, such as unmarried mothers, political dissidents and black and ethnic minorities. This goes some way to explain the paradox we addressed in Chapter 3 about the inverse care law – the bulk of the population may eschew equitable or preferential 'access' to the psychiatric profession.

Second, as we noted above, the elaboration of a contested epistemological field about mental health has not led to professionals inviting lay accounts readily into the field. Professional knowledge is always a meta-account of the patient's view. Even the most client-centred of all forms of professional knowledge, such as that derived from the work of Carl Rogers, entails the professional having a general theory of human functioning and change that forms a frame of possibilities which each client unknowingly enters (Pilgrim 1997). As Bannister (1983) pointed out about psychotherapists and their clients:

> Clearly the relationship between therapist and client is initially neither reciprocal nor equal. If you are the therapist then you and your client are on either side of *your* desk, in your *office*, on *your* patch. Your presence signifies qualifications, expertise and prestige, the client's presence signifies that he or she has 'given in', 'confessed failure'. You as the therapist represent, socially, if not in fact, the healthy ordered life while the client represents sickness and confusion. You prescribe the pattern of the relationship . . . you may decide to be non-directive but, even if so, it will be you that decided to be non-directive. You may negotiate all things but you do so from a position of power. (Bannister 1983: 139)

Bannister is here talking about psychotherapists sitting with their clients (maybe atypically across a desk). Earlier, Haley (1963) had pointed out that classical psychoanalysts put patients in a position, with their feet off the ground and unable to see the professional, which physically underscores the power imbalance. Even in relation to non-directive therapy, arguably the most democratic and least paternalistic of all therapeutic styles, power lurks. Haley noted that it is very difficult for a client to get the better of someone who agrees with them all the time (Rogers' 'accurate empathy').

In relation to our concern here about unequal power, clients are arguably disempowered by the type of knowledge-differential common to all interactions between experts (lawyers, educators, doctors, psychologists, social workers, etc.) and non-experts. There is an axiomatic point which could be made, then, that expertise in all its forms is a ubiquitous source of disempowerment, a point taken to its limits by anti-professional critiques (e.g., Illich 1975). In the case of the psychotherapies, some have argued that it is so riven with the abuse of power that clients may be well advised to struggle on with their mental health problems without the ministrations of professionals (Masson 1988). An additional complication in the case of mental health work is that experts often also have delegated coercive power (see Chapter 3).

Psychiatric knowledge and individualisation

In the next chapter, we will be examining biological treatments. As a prelude in this chapter, it is relevant to mention the causal or aetiological assumptions which underpin them as part of a discussion about psychiatric knowledge individualising madness and misery and closing off the social context from consideration. Biodeterminism may involve both genetic and environmental factors in its assumptions. Brain disease (potentially) can be acquired from injury or infection and at any point from *in utero* onwards, and so can be subject to environmental variation. Environmental variables are patterned by social and spatial determinants. By contrast, genetic hypotheses are unambiguous attributions about biologically fixed sub-populations (families), independent of their spatial or social features. Whilst the notion of 'biological' does not necessarily narrowly imply 'genetic', the *eugenic* legacy and version of biodeterminism dating back to Victorian psychiatry has had a disproportionate impact on psychiatric reasoning.

The eugenic bias of early psychiatry has strong resonances today but reached its apotheosis in the Nazi period. The genetic work of Rudin and Kallman in Germany during that time is still cited favourably by modern-day biological psychiatrists, even if their political mentors and values are conveniently lost to history (see Chapter 6). The recent orthodoxy in psychiatry now centres upon a stress-vulnerability theory. This asserts that the proneness to madness is (or is probably) genetically inherited and the vulnerability to its manifestation in florid symptoms and social dysfunction is thus produced by social stressors in the family and from elsewhere. This is why we noted above that biological psychiatry virtually excludes social reasoning. Not only is social stress reduced to a triggering role but it is invoked as a reason why genetic assertions about causality are logically incontrovertible. The logic is that if all stressed populations (say, combatants or poor people) are subjected to the same level of psychological threat or pressure, why do only some of them become mentally disordered? This point is central to the work of Guze discussed now.

The eugenic tradition of nineteenth-century European psychiatry continued to resonate strongly a century later across the Atlantic, even if modified by the concession to triggering social stressors just noted. In a highly cited paper, given at the Institute of Psychiatry in London, Samuel Guze, Head of Psychiatry at Washington University, states assuredly that:

> what is called psychopathology *is* the manifestation of disordered processes in various brain systems that mediate psychological functions ... By taking into consideration genetic codes and epigenetic development, guided and shaped by broad-ranging environmental influences, only some of which are now recognised and understood, biology *clearly offers* the *only* comprehensive scientific basis for psychiatry just *as it does for the rest of medicine*. (Guze 1989: 317–18, emphasis added)

This quote from Guze highlights points we made earlier about premature certainty and arrogance masking uncertainty and ignorance. Note that the brain is not merely put forward as a possible explanation. It is considered to be *the* explanation – signed, sealed and delivered already by scientific psychiatry. In fact, Guze has no definitive evidence that disordered brains reliably explain disordered functioning (any more than psychodynamic writers have any definitive evidence about their developmental hypotheses). The words 'clearly offers' and 'only' are logically indefensible.

Versions of this taken-for-granted certainty about genetically shaped neurological or neurophysiological processes pepper the writings of biological psychiatrists (Ross and Pam 1995). They lead to junior psychiatrists learning biodeterminism 'by assumption', because trainees are rarely encouraged to reflect critically about the views of their seniors, at least about epistemological tenets (Kemker and Khadivi 1995). Biological certainty is captured in Gerard's phrase 'no twisted thought without a twisted molecule' (Abood 1960) or by 'strange people strange substances' (van Praag 1977). These types of assumption permeate the psychiatric tradition which young doctors begin to inhabit, contribute to and reproduce.

Guze reveals the professional process of a bid for pre-eminent legitimacy on behalf of his profession. His phrase, 'as it does for the rest of medicine', is the key here, with psychiatry still desperate to be accepted as a legitimate medical speciality. Biology has become a political vehicle for the re-professionalisation of the medical speciality of psychiatry and its scientific credibility has consequently suffered. There is little wonder that academic biologists are critical of the logical errors and distorted leaps of faith made by biological psychiatrists about genes and behaviour (Lewontin *et al.* 1984).

Guze's insistence on inherited vulnerability immediately closes off the consideration of external inputs such as poverty, sexual violence, warfare and racism. Instead it limits the focus of psychiatric knowledge to flawed and vulnerable individuals. Whereas social models of madness and misery (and the biopsychosocial model) emphasise open systems reasoning, biological psychiatry produces *closed-systems reasoning* (as do some versions of psychoanalysis). An irony of this criticism is that the distinction between open and closed systems was made in a theory produced within biology and subsequently generalised to social and political science (Luhmann 1982; von Bertalanffy 1968; Wilden 1972). This irony highlights that biology does not have to be cast in the reductionist role favoured by many psychiatrists. Indeed, the clearest exposition of the biopsychosocial model draws explicitly on the tenets of general systems theory (Engel 1980).

What closed systems reasoning does is warrant one form of reality and exclude others. Once the brain and inherited vulnerability have been privileged, a set of important and legitimate open questions (for example, about primary environmental causality and the social negotiation of deviance) are shut down. The matter has been 'pre-emptively construed', to use a term offered by Kelly (1955) – hence our note above about psychiatrists 'learning by assumption'.

The premature certainty of professional knowledge is part of what Boyne (1990), discussing the work of Derrida, calls the 'dishonest certitude that informs the tradition of Western thought'. Unfortunately what this certitude has done is provoke nihilistic relativism and anti-realism in postmodern social science about mental health issues (Rogers and Pilgrim 2001). There has also been a tendency on the part of sociologists from varying theoretical backgrounds to reject biology (Benton 1991). Thus, a political dynamic between academic disciplines in medicine and social science, in which they are ignorant of or hostile to one another and therefore 'talk past' each other, has attended the development of psychiatric knowledge.

Reflecting on the work of Guze and others, Clare (1999), the champion of an even handed biopsychosocial approach we introduced at the start of the chapter, poses a cautionary question:

> As mental hospital gives way to acute district general hospital and community facilities, are the psychological aspects of disease being reabsorbed within the very core of medicine or is psychiatry slowly being filtered and the social domains it has for two centuries so painstakingly valued and endorsed being remorsely discarded? (Clare 1999: 111)

What Clare takes for granted in the caution is that his profession has consistently and collectively understood, valued and properly integrated the non-biological aspects of its work. This may reflect a mistaken belief in the minds of Clare and other champions of the biopsychosocial model. They may confuse the logical and political merits of their preferred integrative approach with its assumed presence in routine psychiatric practice.

Although the holistic tradition upheld by the likes of Meyer and Engel in North America and Henderson, Gillespie and Clare in Britain offered a persuasive rescue package to their profession, in the wake of anti-psychiatry, with their 'portmanteau model', by no means all their colleagues heeded their call. Indeed, currently the position of Guze may more clearly reflect the aspirations of most psychiatrists working in beleaguered services with their medical authority under threat (Samson 1995). The confidence of Guze and other academic psychiatrists in their medical mandate about madness and distress is reflected in the overwhelming preference of psychiatric practitioners for physical treatments in State-provided mental health services, with psychotherapy being reduced to a 'speciality' within the profession rather than an integral part of everyday clinical practice.

The triumphalism of Guze and other biological psychiatrists who proudly own the term 'medical model' (rather than use it as a term of contempt about an unfounded and logically flawed biological reductionism) (Guze and Helzer 1985) has been reinforced by the revision of the North American diagnostic system. Below we cite two leading writers about DSM-IV, the most recent version of the Diagnostic and Statistical Manual (DSM). The diagnostic emphasis under DSM is one of neutrality about aetiology. The main thrust of DSM is not to champion biology as an academic discipline but to champion medicine as a profession:

DSM-III was a landmark in the development of psychiatric classification, drawing on the best available research from the preceding
decades and placing psychiatry *firmly back in the medical model* of
basing treatment decisions on diagnosis. (Blacker and Tsuang 1999: 70,
emphasis added)

The notion of 'going back' to medicine to endorse a medical
model of mental disorder, criticised by internal critics such as
Fernando and celebrated by re-professionalisers like Blacker and
Tsuang, is indicative of a legitimacy crisis in psychiatry. Critics and
conservatives agree on the existence of the phenomenon – the issue
is not about whether psychiatry is being re-medicalised but the reasons why. The latter must lie in the points made by Fernando. The
profession has, in the last thirty years, developed a siege mentality,
with some good reason as we noted earlier, given its aggregating
range of internal and external critics.

According to some sociological analysts, the pre-eminent position
of psychiatry in the mental health industry is now fatally wounded
and its dominance is fragmenting (Samson 1995). If it is not in
terminal decline, it is certainly a recurring focus of disappointment in
its recipients and distrust in the wider culture of medicine. Psychiatry
is not popular among new medical graduates and, in the NHS in
Britain, its acute recruitment crisis is becoming a prolonged structural defect in mental health services.

Whilst the eugenic roots of modern psychiatric biodeterminism
created the most clear-cut version of individualisation by placing
the causes of mental abnormality unambiguously inside individual
bodies, psychoanalytical competitors also have made a similar
contribution. Freud's original theories were developed in relation to
individuals from a particular social background. His preferred
practice and that of the bulk of his followers was of individual treatment. Moreover, his original theory was based upon a hydraulic
version of the mind – a dynamic system of conflicting forces within a
skin-encapsulated closed system which, Freud believed, would
ultimately be explicable in neurological terms. This led to Wolman
(1968) describing Freud as a 'hoped-for-reductionist'.

However, despite Freud's own version of biologism, he opened up
an ambiguous social space in his theory. The inputs to the dynamic
unconscious were from 'triangulated' relationships between the
child and their mother and father – as many have pointed out since,

this assumption of triangulation is not only heterosexist, it may no longer reflect the empirical norm of family life in Western society. Moreover, although the social space created by the Freudian discourse was explored by later psychoanalysts, they offered contradictory accounts about its meaning. Some following Klein, who considered aggression to be instinctually derived and projected outwards by infants, saw tensions, destructiveness and dependency in social organisation as being products of the aggregate outward mapping of individual inner worlds (Bion 1977). In complete contrast, other psychoanalysts argued that mental illness was environmentally determined by problems of sub-standard early mothering (Winnicott 1958), by disruptions in attachments (Bowlby 1951) or by mystifying familial communication systems (Laing and Esterson 1964).

This confusion and ambiguity in psychoanalytical theory is confirmed by the political range of psychoanalytical writing. On the one hand, it was the basis for substantial integrations with Marxism, especially in the Frankfurt School (Slater 1977), on the other, it has been linked to an elite middle-class world of private practice and social conservatism, in which an acceptance of the *status quo* and the psychological maturity of the individual ego are conflated (Chasseguet-Smirgel and Grunberger 1986). Psychoanalysis itself is, thus, a highly uncertain and contested terrain. It is no more capable of delivering a firm unified epistemological footing for medical authority about mental health than is biological psychiatry. More importantly, it converges with the latter in its individualistic assumptions, but with minds not brains being flawed.

Thus, the two dominant psychiatric models during the past hundred years, biodeterminism and psychoanalysis, have been linked to varieties of individualism which have closed off social relationships. Whilst it is true that eugenically derived biodeterminism represents the main example of this point, psychoanalysis has not offered itself up as a consistent corrective to methodological individualism within the profession. By and large, clinical psychoanalysis and its spin-off (the psychodynamic psychotherapies) have reinforced, not challenged, the individualisation of madness and misery.

Normative knowledge and social control

Leaving aside ideological disputes about aetiology, psychiatric treatment has been marshalled in its totality to variants of social control. All sides of the argument – biological, psychodynamic or biopsychosocial – have retained a normative view of mental life. Psychiatric nosology, supported by all camps, has ultimately defined mental abnormality essentially with reference to role–rule failure and social incompetence. The psychotic patient with their mad talk and unintelligible actions offends the social contract of mutual respect and intentional transparency. The paranoid makes rigid and hostile claims about reality which others fail to support. The depressive withdraws from social life and their work and family obligations to various degrees. The anxious person fearfully avoids these obligations. Successful psychiatric treatment restores these varieties of deviance to the fold of a shared moral order. Unsuccessful treatment leaves us with incorrigible madness and chronic neurosis.

Psychiatry and its subordinate and competing professions have offered both voluntary *and* coercive solutions to role–rule failure and social incompetence. The psychotherapies actively sought and gratefully received are stylised conversations which, if successful, offer pay-offs to the sufferer and the social order they inhabit. Drug treatments taken voluntarily offer the hope of cure-while-you-wait, with little need for personal struggle or existential reflection. For the mad, drugs can be imposed against their consent under the State's blessing of mental health legislation. Thus, the mental health industry, including interventions in primary health care settings, in the first instance, produces conformity in the same way in which Parsons described physical medicine, through a consensual negotiation of entrance to and departure from the sick role. If this fails, it deploys a variant of coercive policing by tidying up 'residual deviance' (Scheff 1966), given that all psychiatric crises are social crises, in which 'something has to be done' (Bean 1980). Voluntary and coercive control coexist in psychiatric practice at any particular time about whole patient populations and they shift fluidly over time in the 'management' of individuals.

Thus, when any person with a mental health problem presents themselves or is presented by others to psychiatric attention, they enter a social space in which an inequality of power operates. The codification of this unequal interaction by professional knowledge mirrors (usually implicitly) the normative concerns of the social order both parties inhabit. Critics of psychiatric knowledge have sometimes focused on disputed, marginal or atypical cases where social deviance is being unfairly medicalised (e.g., homosexuality being classified as a mental disorder or political dissidents being diagnosed and treated by psychiatrists in the former USSR). However, this type of critique is limited and potentially misleading, as it may imply that psychiatry is not normative in its mundane working assumptions and the intentions of its daily practice (Conrad and Schneider 1985). The codification of madness as 'schizophrenia' or misery as 'clinical depression' are regular cases in point. Mad people break rules and miserable people withdraw from their roles. When it is successful, psychiatry reverses these social processes.

As we noted in Chapters 3 and 4, psychiatry is part of a broad apparatus of social regulation. The voluntaristic wing of this control overlaps with the wider healing role of medicine about warranting entrance to and departure from the sick role. Its coercive wing overlaps with policing and the penal system. The most obvious form of this is in relation to mentally disordered offenders (inhabiting secure mental health services). Its less obvious form is in relation to non-offenders detained under mental health legislation, such as civil sections of the British Mental Health Act of 1983. Our argument here, for now, is not whether psychiatry should or should not fulfil a social control role, but that the role exists.

Above, we noted that the normative nature of psychiatric knowledge may be implicit for its practitioners. One aspect of 'learning by assumption' in psychiatric training is that the work of the profession is about treating people with mental illness, who may, as a result of their lack of attributed insight and adjudged threat to self or others, require paternalistic medical care. This assumption about warranted medical paternalism may lead to psychiatrists having little habitual sense of their social control role. However, the evidence for the role lies in the concerns we noted earlier in Chapter 3 about the paradoxical position concerning psychiatry and the inverse care law. It also lies in the hostility expressed by black people about psychiatry's disproportionate interest in their detention and treatment (Francis 1988).

Knowledge and status differentials

Up to now, in this chapter, we have focused upon psychiatric knowledge because of its dominance. The latter has had to be maintained (over patients and competing professionals) and so the knowledge-base of psychiatry has interwoven confident knowledge-claims with confidence about its leadership role in the field of mental health.

However, psychiatry is only one of several professions which are sometimes now called the 'psy complex'. Others, such as mental health nursing, psychiatric social work and clinical psychology, are part of the mental health industry. Nursing and social work as semi-professions have not defined a clear and separate identity for themselves from medicine. They either follow the contours of psychiatric knowledge or occasionally oppose it (Goldie 1978). Clinical psychology, a much smaller profession, is peculiar in that its academic status as a discipline is more clear cut. Indeed, medicine is not an academic discipline but a constellation of contributions from academic departments (from anatomy to sociology) harnessed for a *vocational* goal of medical practice. Medical training is rarely pre-occupied with epistemological issues but instead emphasises professional competence and confidence in clinical settings managing a range of problematic populations. One of these groups is distressed or mad people, whose difficulties for themselves or others are then reconstructed as psychiatric illnesses or mental disorder by professional interventions (de Swann 1990).

The issue of status differentials (another connotation of the notion of inequality) has a double significance. First, the relationship of mental health to physical health, can be considered in terms of its constituent professions and service delivery systems. In Britain, the policy salience of mental health suggests that, at least at the level of government policy, it fairs well. For example, improving mental health was one of five main targets set by Tony Blair in the NHS plan announced in 2000. Also, in the previous year, the National Service Framework for Mental Health was the first to be announced as part of a series of service frameworks, indicating something about its political importance (see Chapter 4).

However, this political salience may reflect a concern about risk and scandals which politicians are keen to avoid, rather than a clear and sophisticated rationale about mental health policy. An example of this is that for such a wide range of problems (from anxiety states and depression through to psychosis and personality disorder), the main outcome indicator at governmental level has been crude (the reduction of suicide levels). As we noted in the previous chapter, not only is suicide a highly limited indicator that has little or nothing to say about the bulk of mental health problems most of the time, it may not even be an indicator of mental health problems at all. It may, for some people, represent a logical and existentially meaningful form of action. This crudity is not evident in the domain of physical health policy, where a long list of specific outcomes is identified for particular patient populations.

Second, within the mental health industry the existence of professions competing with one another and challenging medical dominance has implications for interdisciplinary relationships and, thus, the efficiency and coherence of mental health services. This is a complex and contradictory field. For example, whilst the dominant profession, psychiatry, is now losing its authority to, or credibility in the eyes of, other disciplines and it remains a lowly medical speciality with a recruitment crisis, this is not the case for all mental health work. Clinical psychology is highly attractive to psychology graduates. What recruitment problems exist in mental health services is a function of a training bottleneck, with applications for postgraduate training currently outstripping supply of places by six to one. Whilst the status of psychiatry may have diminished over time, the opposite has been true for clinical psychology.

Moreover, the knowledge-base of clinical psychology is itself contradictory. At times, it has been parasitical upon psychiatric knowledge when conducting randomised controlled trials on psychological treatments for diagnostic categories, such as 'schizophrenia' or 'depression' (e.g., Blackburn *et al.* 1981; Tarrier *et al.* 1993). At other times, it has advocated a radically different (single-symptom) approach and rejected the validity of psychiatric diagnoses (Bentall *et al.* 1988; Boyle 1990).

The most dramatic turning point in the political relationship between clinical psychology and psychiatry in Britain occurred when Hans Eysenck presented a paper to the Royal Medico-Psychological Association (now the Royal College of Psychiatrists) arguing that the authority for the treatment of neurosis should be handed over from psychiatry to psychology (Eysenck 1958). He subsequently reinforced this point by arguing for a division of labour, with psychology dealing with neurosis and biological psychiatry with madness (Eyesenck 1975). In the early days of the profession of clinical psychology at the Institute of Psychiatry, Eysenck had maintained a totally different position. He had previously reasoned that psychologists should be disinterested scientists assessing and formulating problems, and that treatment entailed value driven goals. Consequently, in this first phase the treatment role was eschewed (Eysenck 1949).

The consequence of the bid for legitimacy from clinical psychology to erode the therapeutic mandate of medicine was of prolonged antagonism between the two professions (Pilgrim and Treacher 1992). By the late 1970s, this culminated in psychology being granted independence from psychiatric dominance in the NHS (Trethowan 1977). The irritation evoked in psychiatrists at the time by this competition is exemplified sardonically here by Clare (1979):

> As far as clinical psychology is concerned, it is in the midst of clarifying the precise terms and conditions of its takeover bid for those assets of Psychiatry Limited which it believes more properly belong to it.

Given that Clare was at the same time championing the bio-psychosocial model in his profession, his statement strongly suggests that such a model was about expanding a psychiatric knowledge-base to retain medical authority. The model has not been about giving epistemological power over to other professions but an integrationist attempt to justify traditional medical dominance.

The uneasy relationship between psychology and psychiatry has been evident, if to a lesser extent, between all the mental health professions. This has led to recurring time consuming disputes and non-cooperation in mental health services. The rhetoric of 'multi-disciplinary' teamwork has witnessed a less persuasive reality at times, with teamwork being a focus of conflict and threat about the erosion of unidisciplinary confidence (Onyett *et al.* 1994).

'Power is knowledge': the challenge of lay knowledge

Our discussion so far illuminates the way in which the notion of 'need' in relation to mental health varies according to competing professional perspectives and knowledge. In simple terms, psychiatrists and other mental health professionals produce clinical notions of need, whereas lay people use other criteria. We have seen in Chapters 3 and 4 how, during service contact, these worldviews meet and coincide or collide. In recent times, there have been policy attempts to reconcile divergent views of need. For example, a patient perspective is increasingly accepted as a necessary element in the evaluation of service provision and quality assurance. In the UK, recent government mental health policy has emphasised that the users should find services accessible, acceptable and appropriate and that these quality indicators should be considered alongside more traditional outcomes, such as efficiency.

This quality assurance trend has focused mental health service audits and evaluations on patient satisfaction. Whilst this approach has obvious merit (compared to not asking service users at all), a surface snapshot cannot reveal a deeper view from patients based upon their cumulative experience. Moreover, attempts at incorporating an excluded party may still fail to recognise the inimical differences between a clinical and user perspective of need in the configuration and delivery of services. The latter have a long history of being defined and run according to clinical norms.

Previously, we have pointed to different ways in which professionally dominated knowledge excludes a valid user viewpoint (Rogers *et al.* 1993). Whilst it is now included in health policy, it is usually established and legitimised only in so far as it conforms to orthodox means of measuring and improving quality in services. In practice, the danger is of an increasingly reified and restricted set of 'user outcomes' which actually centre on professional imperatives.

For example, it is increasingly common for users to be asked about their understanding of the advantages and disadvantages of working arrangements of mental health services, e.g., the 'Care Programme Approach' or the 'Mental Health Register'. Such measures are designed by policy-makers for implementation by mental health professionals. This particular focus on user outcomes has emerged over the last two decades at a time when the language of markets, contracts and consumers has played a significant role in the commissioning and delivery of mental health services. However, this type of 'user outcomes' focus contrasts starkly with instances when users are given a licence to *define* as well as implement an agenda about need and its implied response.[1]

The MHUM (mental health user movement) has acted as a countervailing force to experts, control and production of knowledge. To an extent, psychiatric patients' construction of knowledge is both engendered and constantly reinforced by their experience of illness and by their contact with professional services. This is evident in the way in which the 'Hearing Voices' network run by users describes what 'voice hearing is about':

'Hearing voices' has been regarded by psychiatry as an auditory hallucination and in many cases a symptom of schizophrenia. However, not everyone who hears voices has a diagnosis of schizophrenia. There are conflicting theories about why people hear voices from psychiatrists, psychologists and voice hearers. Although the network is open to many diverse opinions *and we accept all and respect the individual explanation of the person who hears voices*. (http://www.hearing-voices.org.uk/about.htm)

The version of a lay voice inside the domains of services provision and the socialisation of mental health professionals may obscure another, that of an 'alternative' lay knowledge which has not only challenged the assumptions of professional knowledge but has provided a connection with the broader everyday life experiences of individuals. The work of Estroff (1981) in the US and Barham and Hayward (1991) has highlighted the wider meaning of mental distress in the lives of patients discharged to live in the community. In particular, they illuminate attempts by individuals to engender or sustain an identity as a person rather than a mental patient. Drawing on individual experiences, some unique some shared, a collective identity had emerged from the activities of the MHUM. In turn, the latter has formed the basis of collective action (Rogers and Pilgrim 1991). This has not happened in a social vacuum. Rather, the emergence of the 'personalised' voice of the mental patient has been formulated in a dialogical relationship with wider influences operating in the health and social care field (Crossley and Crossley 2001). Mental health groups have sought to assert both the legitimacy of experiential knowledge and their positions as citizens in the face of official responses, which have construed them as self-interested pressure groups (Barnes 1999).

Lay knowledge and resistance

Sources of lay knowledge have also constituted a minority focus of the research agenda about inequalities and mental health. In relation to the management of mental health problems, the power of lay knowledge to act as a counter to professional knowledge is still relatively marginal. Nonetheless, there are significant spaces in the voluntary sector, where user-led programmes have been effective in promoting user conceptualisations of mental health which have acted to compete with professional knowledge (Faulkner 1997). Radical public health approaches to research have also encouraged the expression of lay knowledge about threats to health and, at times, lay knowledge has been privileged over more traditional perspectives. There are examples of 'lay epidemiology' where lay knowledge has been viewed as more advanced than 'experts' in claims about causal relationships between pathogenic social conditions and ill health (e.g., Brown 1992). In relation to the genesis of mental health problems, the focus on user defined concepts points to understanding conceptualisations of mental health differently. For example, Davidson (2000) has recently pointed up the relevance of recognising social and spatial aspects, alongside the individual construction of 'lived space', from accounts provided by sufferers of agoraphobia. Lay knowledge is seen as directly emancipatory in addressing the marginal status of those diagnosed with a mental health problem. For an example of this, we can return to what the Hearing Voices Network has to say about bringing about change:

> People who hear voices and their families and friends can gain greater benefits from de-stigmatising the experience, leading to a greater tolerance and understanding. This can be achieved through promoting more positive explanations which give people a more positive framework for developing their own ways of coping and raising awareness about the experience in society as a whole. (www.hearing-voices.org.uk/abootu.htm)

There are areas of lay and professional knowledge which coalesce. Constructs may appear on the surface to be used in a way which describes a common phenomenon. However, there are difficulties in finding an appropriate alternative terminology to that introduced by a medical model. Lay people have a rich experiential knowledge of personal well-being (what might be called mental health) but the expression of this state and its disruption may not be easy for them to express. Inchoate feelings may inhibit such expression, as described here by one person we interviewed in a project about the promotion of mental health:

> It's a very difficult thing to explain [mental health] because you don't go around thinking about it most of the time ... things are just chugging along really. Then it can strike you out of the blue. Suddenly you realise you are not coping, and its different from being ill physically because somehow you aware you are not feeling too good. I mean with both [physical and mental health] you've got ill and not ill but most of the time with physical health you're somewhere in between. But with mental health you're just not aware what's going on until it's too late. (Rogers and Pilgrim 1997: 28)

Despite the difficulties of expressing the experience of mental health problems, a facet of user knowledge is the relatively free-flowing connectedness between social and personal events and the feelings and emotions experienced by individuals. The lay emphasis on social stressors in aetiology, when talking about maintaining mental health, and the relevance of social forces in influencing the experience of living with a mental health problem point to the need to develop interventions which focus on aspects of maintaining and enhancing a positive sense of personal identity and citizenship. Lay constructs as well as participation can be built into the philosophy and delivery of service as innovations in 'community development' and user-led initiatives show. However, the extent to which mainstream services are able to engage with and incorporate models of care based on lay knowledge is likely to be limited as long as professional interests, models and practices are prioritised within service provision.

Conclusion

This chapter has drawn attention to the relationship between the knowledge-base of the mental health professions, particularly psychiatry, and power in a number of senses. First, knowledge is bound up with gaining and retaining power over colleagues in competing professions and patients. Second, knowledge-claims warrant or disallow a consideration of the social context of power relationships. Third, knowledge-in-action within mental health work is bound up with social regulation and therefore is part of the reproduction of pre-existing social hierarchies and forms of social organisation – it has a normative function. Fourth, *both* biological *and* psychological bodies of knowledge within mental health work have individualised the social by their respective versions of reductionism. Finally, we have considered the emergence of lay knowledge as a competing paradigm to professionalised knowledge about mental health. Knowledge based on personal experience provides a closer fit with the social conditions and personal experiences which give rise to mental health problems. The unequal structural position of users and professionals is likely to inhibit the full potential that lay knowledge has in developing policies and practices which tackle social exclusion and the inequities associated with mental health.

8

Biological treatments: a case of imposed equality

Introduction

It is unusual for those who receive a diagnosis of mental illness to remain completely untreated. The great bulk of patients receive biological interventions, usually psychotropic drugs, occasionally ECT and, very rarely, psychosurgery. Such treatments are also routinely prescribed alongside talking treatments (Olfson and Pincus 1999). Thus, virtually everyone with a mental health problem has access to biological treatments or may have them imposed.

Early studies of social class differences (Hollingshead and Redlich 1958) demonstrated that lower-class people were less likely to receive talking treatments and more likely to receive drugs and ECT (see next chapter). Also, the study of uneven medication prescription compared to the availability and administration of other forms of treatment has been used as one means of illuminating potentially racist practices within mental health services (Littlewood and Lipsedge 1995). Thus, although we argue in this chapter that biological treatments are a form of imposed equality, it is also important to emphasise that there are also inequalities in access to alternatives to this imposition.

It could be pointed out, in relation to people with physical illnesses, that drug treatments are not simply accessed or declined by patients. Some medications are not prescribed equitably (e.g., beta-interferon for the treatment of muscular sclerosis) or they are medically regulated to minimise iatrogenic effects (e.g., in the UK antibiotics are not sold over the counter). Additionally, access to drug treatments are governed, to some extent, by the financial resources of patients.[1] This might suggest that psychiatric prescribing is not unusual within medicine. However, a particular feature of psychiatric drugs is that there is greater scope for norms about the negotiation of medication to be shaped much more by third party interests and by the threat of coercion. In physical medicine, with a more consistent ethos of voluntary contact and choice, and growing consumerist norms filtering into patient relationships with health services, professional practice is perennially subject to modification by patient demand . Thus, whilst a neat divide does not exist between psychiatric and non-psychiatric prescribing to adults, they are significantly different.

In relation to children, medical practitioners are more cautious about prescribing psychotropic drugs. Indeed, sometimes professionals are a brake upon the enthusiasm of some parents with 'hyperactive' children for medication. However, despite this relative medical reticence, the prescription rate of psychiatric drugs for children has increased in the last ten years. For example, studies in the USA confirmed that between 1990 and 1996 the prescription of methylphenidate (trade name: Ritalin) doubled for pre-school children, with a significant increase also in the prescription to this age-group of fluoxetine (trade name: Prozac) (Gottlieb 2000). Reviews of the field demonstrate that every class of psychotropic agent used in adult psychiatry (including lithium and anti-psychotics) is also deployed in child psychiatry (Campbell *et al.* 1999).

If biological treatments are so commonplace, does this mean that they are popular? The answer to this question is both 'yes' and 'no'. Biological treatments are certainly popular with medical practitioners. Most psychiatrists are chemotherapists and psychotherapy is a 'speciality' (i.e., a minor pursuit) in the profession. In primary care, the staple response to common forms of mental distress for GPs is the prescription of antidepressants and anxiolytics (anti-anxiety agents). However, drugs generally are not as popular with patients as with professionals. The mental health service users' movement has been critical of biological treatments and has continued to demand greater access to psychological alternatives. User opposition is particularly strong in relation to ECT and psychosurgery.

In order to understand this disjuncture between professional popularity and service user unpopularity, we need to unpack the perspectives of the two interest groups. We also need to understand other sustaining factors, such as the function of mental health services and the compatibility of biological interventions with this

function. Also, because chemotherapy is not just a therapeutic transaction between a prescriber and a receiver but also a technology
which is produced for profit by a third party (the pharmaceutical
companies), the socio-economic dynamic that the free market brings
into mental health work requires consideration.

This chapter will consider:

- Biodeterminism and medical dominance in the mental health
  industry
- The compatibility of biological treatments and coercive control
- The role of the pharmaceutical industry
- User opposition to biological treatments.

Any understanding of biological dominance in models of mental
health work has to start with a recognition of medical dominance.
Historically, had the medical profession not established its dominance in State-delegated powers to manage madness, then we would
now be faced with a different way of understanding and organising
mental health work. Medical dominance is by no means fixed and
irrevocable, however. In the latter part of the twentieth century, the
capacity of a narrow medical approach to be sustained was being
undermined from several directions: the failure of a century of
expensive medical research to deliver the biological explanation for
madness; a hostile opposition movement from disaffected patients;
competing bids for legitimacy by non-medical mental health workers, such as nurses and clinical psychologists; and dissent from within
the ranks of psychiatry itself. Moreover, the legitimation crisis of
medicine is not limited to psychiatry as a specialism. All medical
knowledge has been contested increasingly by lay people and
competing professionals (Gabe *et al*. 1994; Haug 1988).

This cultural point about a somatic emphasis and biological treatments is a caution against the temptation to explain the pre-eminent
role of drug treatments merely in terms of drug company profit-
seeking. The latter is important, as we shall see later, but it is not the
whole story – the epistemological emphasis in psychiatry's view of
madness and misery needs to be understood as well. The medical
profession with its biological emphasis and the pharmaceutical
industry with its appetite for profit have had a collusive, symbiotic
and synergistic relationship, so they need to be considered in tandem.
However, an indication about the biological preference of the

psychiatric profession operating independently of drug company influence is the continued use of non-drug treatments such as ECT and psychosurgery. Also, as we note later, biodeterminism well pre-dated the growing influence of the pharmaceutical industry.

The compatibility of biological treatments and coercive control

The emphasis upon biodeterminism and its link to medical tradition touched upon an important historical springboard for the profession of psychiatry – the management of madness. Within institutional psychiatry, mechanical restraints eventually gave way to chemical restraints. The formal nomenclature which is still used today to describe psychiatric drugs is telling – 'sedatives', 'hypnotics' and 'tranquillisers'. These words are, of course, highly ambiguous. They can invoke images of the calming of distress and the sufferer's respite from distraught agitation. The other connotation is more repressive. The drugs may sedate, hypnotise or tranquillise a person out of a level of sensibility required to function autonomously or optimally.

When drugs are received gratefully and voluntarily and are experienced as helpful – the antidepressant which lifts a black mood or the anxiolytic which calms the distress of an over-anxious person – then the first connotation above finds an embodied reality for the patient and in the helping relationship with their treating physician. However, the roots of psychiatry primarily were not about this type of social transaction but about the management of madness. The latter took place in a context of enforced segregation from society. Initially this meant that all lunatics were detained forcibly ('certified'). With increasing public concern about the unfair detention of the sane, this blanket rule about certification gave way to a more measured and discriminating form of mental health law (after 1930 in Britain) in which only a minority of patients were coercively detained. By the 1980s, in Britain only about 8 per cent of psychiatric patients were hospitalised against their will, at least according to official records.

However, as we have seen in previous chapters, the coercive role of psychiatry has not diminished in a linear fashion in the last hundred years. Biological treatments, especially drugs, are relevant for this picture of the recurring and increasingly coercive role of psychiatry in society. They can be administered involuntarily. Indeed, via mental health law the State does not only delegate powers to mental health professionals to *detain* mad people, it also gives them lawful powers to impose treatments on reluctant bodies.

Talking treatments are much more problematic in this regard, as they require some reasonable level of patient cooperation. Indeed some therapists argue that talking treatment in secure settings violates a fundamental starting premise of psychotherapy – voluntarism. By contrast, drugs are impersonal and so they can be administered impersonally. The patient refusing to swallow can be forcibly injected. Moreover, within involuntary settings other, more coercive, spaces often exist – rooms dedicated to the seclusion of individual patients. In these settings, patients are often not merely isolated, they are also forcibly injected with tranquillisers, sometimes with fatal consequences (HMSO 1992). Given that black patients are placed in secure environments more often and perceived to be more dangerous than white counterparts with the same symptoms, they are also more likely to suffer this fate (Noble and Rodger 1989).

Probably the most telling manifestation of the coercive potential of major tranquillisers and their prescribers is that they have been used on a whole range of populations which are not, by medical criteria, psychotic. These include prisoners, people with learning difficulties, disruptive children and agitated older people. This explicit use of tranquillisation for non-psychotic deviant populations has been linked to an ambivalent professional ethical position. For example, on the one hand, Western psychiatrists condemned the use of coercive treatment in response to political dissidence in the old Soviet Union (Bloch and Reddaway 1977). On the other hand, some Western psychiatrists are enthusiastic about the use of major tranquillisers with children who are hyperactive or have learning difficulties (Campbell *et al.* 1999). The latter extensive review is described by the authors as 'critical'. However, the text reveals that this word is used in a scientific, not ethical or political, sense. Evidence is reviewed about the safety and efficacy of anti-psychotic medication with children but at no point do the authors question the wisdom of their use with this group, the particular problems of informed consent, or the extended role of the drugs in quelling challenging or disruptive behaviour (for example, in relation to learning difficulties, autism and hyperactivity).

This mixed professional response, from outrage to enthusiasm, suggests that psychiatrists consider that their role as agents of coercive social control is legitimate in some circumstances but not in others (or that the profession is divided in its commitment to paternalism). Thus, the coercive service function of psychiatry is an important dimension to consider if we are analysing the enduring dominance of biological treatment. The latter is functionally available for a coercive role. To use the modern discourse of managerialism, it is 'fit for purpose'. As with medical knowledge and drug company profit, it is not *the* explanation for the dominance of biological interventions but it is one contributory factor in a multifactorial picture.

The role of the pharmaceutical industry

A confirmation that the biological preferences of psychiatry preceded the supportive role of the drug companies is that the profession had existed for around a hundred years using only a very limited range of medicines. The early limited range of chemical agents included bromides, barbiturates, opiates and a few sedatives such as scopolamine. The capability of these options was so poor that they were regularly augmented by physical restraints and interventions, such as baths and wet packs, psychosurgery and shock treatment (induced by convulsant drugs or electricity). Of these augmenting methods, ECT and psychosurgery remain today.

In the 1950s, a 'pharmacological revolution' is said to have taken place, with the introduction of lithium salts (for mood disorders), chlorpromazine (the first major anti-psychotic agent) and two classes of antidepressant (monoamine oxidase inhibitors and the tricyclic drugs). By 1960, the industry was producing drugs for all the major psychiatric diagnostic categories including, in that year, the first benzodiazepine anxiolytic (Librium). By the mid-1970s, part of the critique of biological psychiatry included an analysis of the work of the drug companies over that twenty-year period of 'revolution'. Their role in accounting for the enduring dominance of physical treatments was highlighted by several critics but most evocatively by Klass (1975) in *There's Gold in Them Thar Pills*.

The main ideological divide before and after the 'pharmacological revolution' of the 1950s relates to the professional agenda that paralleled the economic one of the drug companies. Before 1950, drugs were only seen as a secondary and symptom reduction adjunct to psychiatric treatment in hospital. They sedated and tranquillised. After the 1950s, the terminology of the drugs now reflected curative pretensions. Thus, they were increasingly classified and designated as 'antidepressants' or 'anti-psychotics' implying that they actually cured mental illness (Moncrieff 2002). Psychiatrists were content to promote such a therapeutic optimisim (or arrogance) – so, too, were the drug companies.

As Baruch and Treacher (1978) point out in their review of the historical development of the use of drugs in psychiatry, some prominent academic psychiatrists considered that ward activity and occupational therapy might produce the same rehabilitative impact as the (then) new neuroleptic drugs. Moreover, at the end of the 1950s, when the first neuroleptics (also called 'major tranquillisers') were introduced on a mass scale, early reports suggested that they had more impact in a context in which patients were understimulated in poor custodial regimes. To confirm this, several studies then and since have confirmed that major tranquillisers have their maximal impact when used in combination with psychosocial interventions (including skills training and forms of family management). Despite this, many psychotic patients find that the major tranquillisers are essentially the only treatment offered to them on a regular basis.

At the end of the 1950s, at their inception, the neuroleptics were given in low doses but gradually the average prescribed dose increased. By the 1970s, disabling mega-dosing (large doses) and drug combinations (polypharmacy) were commonplace in psychiatry (Hemmenki 1977; Warner 1985). In part, this was due to aggressive marketing by the drug companies. Their sales representatives argued that high doses produced more therapeutic impact on psychotic symptoms. The extent of prescribing is indicated by official government records. For example, the psychotropic proportion of the NHS drugs bill rose from 17 per cent in 1984 to 24 per cent in 1992. Despite the regular appearance of iatrogenic problems, the 1970s did not stem the upward trend in mega-dosing. One 12-year longitudinal study in the USA found that dose levels of neuroleptics nearly doubled after 1973 (Segal *et al.* 1992). This occurred during a period when the psychopharmacological literature failed to support the prescribing assumption about a dose-response relationship.

Bearing in mind the professional susceptibility to embrace physical treatments, psychiatrists tried old and new drugs in various combinations and dose levels when treating madness in the last quarter of the twentieth century. However, drug treatments were also showing signs of nemesis. First the benzodiazepines (minor tranquillisers) became discredited and then more and more doubts were cast (mainly by patient critics, see below) upon the credibility of the major tranquillisers because of their disabling and sometimes life threatening effects. These difficulties for the drug companies did not temper their enthusiasm. They merely developed and promoted alternatives during the 1980s and 1990s. Benzodiazepines were displaced, partially by multi-purpose antidepressants or other drugs. In low doses, antidepressants have an anxiolytic effect, as do low-dose neuroleptics. Antidepressants, which were toxic and used successfully by suicidal patients, were replaced by less lethal ones. The neuroleptics were joined by new, 'atypical', anti-psychotic agents.

The resilience of drug company activity in the wake of adverse opinion, evidence and experience had already given the industry confidence. For example, at the very time that the neuroleptics were being hailed as wonder drugs, another psychotropic agent, Contergan (thalidomide), was marketed extensively by the German company Chemi Grunenthal. Thalidomide led to the birth of over six thousand children with severe physical defects and was withdrawn. What is significant about the thalidomide case is that it did not undermine medical confidence in psychotropic drug treatment and it clearly did not dent the confidence of the drug companies in promoting new psychotropic agents.

Medical practice and drug industry activity were also undiminished in the face of other evidence. For example, it was becoming clear after the 1970s that high average doses of neuroleptics were leading to an iatrogenic pandemic of movement disorders, an adverse effect of neuroleptics involving Parkinsonism, dystonias and tardive dyskinesia or 'TD'. Estimates of iatrogenic TD range from 0.5 per cent to 50 per cent (with a mean of 20 per cent), with controversy surrounding the degree of permanence of the condition (estimates of permanence vary from six months to ten years) (Baldessarini 1999). TD involves involuntary spasms of the facial muscles, entailing grimacing, tongue flicking and eye rolling. Sometimes the facial symptoms of TD extend to the limbs and trunk (tardive dystonia). These iatrogenic symptoms may be painful and are certainly socially disabling, as they create an odd physical presentation, adding to the stigma of being a psychiatric patient. These adverse effects make some patients understandably 'non-compliant', although the latter tends to be attributed in the professional discourse at times with a lack of motivation and insight on the part of patients about their illness.

Brown and Funk (1986), in a review of the TD literature, pointed out that the low social status and passivity of psychotic patients had led to a level of tolerance of prescribing practices which would not be evident in more assertive and less stigmatised groups of patients. Thus, the ability of the psychiatric profession and the drug companies to evade proper accountability has to be placed in the context of the capacity of patients to oppose unwanted treatment practices and for non-patients to pass a view on the management of madness. Moreover, other recurrent adverse effects of neuropletics, such as akathisia (a state of unrelenting inner restlessness) and acute dysphoria (a sudden and frightening drop in mood), mark out the neuroleptics as very 'dirty' drugs.[2]

Cohen (1997), in a review of the neuroleptics literature, points out that only one in three medicated patients fails to relapse and that there is predictable detrimental impact on social functioning in recipients. Cohen concludes that 'the "neuroleptics" near sacred reputation as "anti-psychotics" is equalled only by their record as one of the most behaviourally toxic classes of psychotropic drugs' (Cohen 1997: 201). The newer 'atypical' anti-psychotics have not been without serious side effects, even though they produce fewer movement disorders. For example, one of them, sertindole (trade name: Serdolect), was withdrawn from use in 1998 following reports of cardiac arrhythmias and cardiac arrest being induced in some of its recipients. Another, clozaril (trade name: Clozapine), has been linked to the development of the serious blood disorder, agranulocytosis (see below).

The ultimate toxic effect of neuroleptics entails them inducing acute cardio-toxicity leading to death (Kellam 1987). Such a state is rare but when it occurs it is usually in the wake of intra-muscular injection of the drug, usually in conditions of pre-existing physiological arousal, such as when an angry patient is secluded. Healy (1997) makes the ironical point that chlorpromazine (the first marketed phenothiazine) was originally sold over the counter as an anti-emetic. Had phenothiazines remained only in self-administered pill form, rather than as a medically prescribed injection, they would have killed fewer people. Apart from acute cardio-toxic reactions to injected neuroleptics causing death, it has also been demonstrated that poor prescribing practices (polypharmacy) and poor anticholinergic control lead to raised mortality rates in psychotic patients over a ten-year period (Waddington *et al.* 1998).

Outside the arena of madness, in primary care, another marketing triumph emerged in the late 1980s – the promotion of the new SSRI antidepressants (selective serotonin re-uptake inhibitors). Prozac (first released for public consumption in 1987) is the most famous trade name for this class of drugs, which is marketed in 'me-too' versions by several companies. What was significant about the new antidepressants is that they were being portrayed not only as safe (non-toxic and non-dysphoria-inducing) but also as euphoriants. Whereas the older antidepressants (the monoamine-oxidase inhibitors and tricyclics) only claimed to lift mood in those depressed, the newer drugs were also marketed as non-addictive agents to increase the vitality and efficiency of people who were not depressed. Despite this apparent discovery of a safe new 'happy pill' to enhance our daily domestic and work performances, the SSRIs began to be linked in some recipients with addiction, self-harm and irritable hostility to others. Healy (2000) suggests that SSRI-induced akathisia accounted for one death per week and one suicide attempt *per day* after the launch of Prozac in the UK.

Healy (1997) makes the important point that out of logical necessity the drug companies are the main source of information for medical practitioners and other health workers about drugs, especially about new agents. Even if the medical undergraduate curriculum contains more critical appraisals of psychiatric or other drugs, these can only be about drugs in established use. Moreover, with the limited opportunities for continuous medical education, trained staff have less time to appraise practice (compared to being a full-time student). In these circumstances, there is a tendency for qualified practitioners to become reliant on drug company-supplied information. All psychiatric and GP journals are peppered with advertisements for psychotropic products.

Also, drug promotion has extended to advertising directly to patients. In 1999 in the USA, the drug companies spent US $1.5 billion promoting their wares using 'direct to consumer' methods. Some promotion of this type is about the euphoriant property of the newer antidepressants. For example, in 1999 SmithKline Beecham spent US $30 million on the targeted advertising of Seroxat as a cure for shyness. Drug companies sponsor academic conferences for psychiatrists and they offer money for research projects and journal production. For example, between 1996 and 2000 eighteen drug companies made a joint contribution of US $12 million to research done by the National Alliance for the Mentally Ill (a mental health charity). The funding by drug companies of academic activities in universities has led to accusations of undue covert influences over academic appointments in psychiatry, when profit might be threatened by academic criticism.

When Dr David Healy gave a lecture at Toronto University which pointed out the dangers associated with the newer antidepressants, a consequence of his talk seemed to be that the university withdrew its offer of a professional contract to him. According to newspaper reports (e.g., 'Biller Pill', *The Guardian*, 7 May 2001), this step could only be understood in the light of Toronto receiving drug company funding.

Given the citations we make in this chapter of Healy's work, it was public knowledge, even before the speech, that he took a sceptical view about drug treatment and was known to be critical of both the drug companies and some of the norms of his own profession. The latter include the regular consumption of drug company food and the acceptance of small gifts, not just at conferences, but also at regular local junior medical training. It is currently the norm in the NHS for the drug companies to provide free food for junior psychiatrists and GPs. Thus, medical practice, training and research are highly enmeshed with the activities of the pharmaceutical industry. The latter did not create the biological bias in psychiatric thinking but it certainly reinforces and maintains the historical trend.

User opposition to biological treatments

The sources of user disaffection about physical treatments are multiple:

- First, there is the issue of resented paternalism – prescription is *ipso facto* paternalistic.
- Second, there is a philosophical motif of bioreductionism being offensive to human complexity and sensibility. This moral rejection of biology could be found strongly in the 'anti-psychiatrists', as well as in the later users' movement. It is hardly surprising that many of the leading 'anti-psychiatrists', such as Laing, Cooper and Szasz, were psychotherapists (the competing wing of psychiatric treatment discussed in the next chapter).
- Third, users are understandably sensitive about the iatrogenic effects of treatments, whereas professionals tend to consider adverse

effects only as part of a wider appraisal of cost effectiveness. For example, Finn *et al.* (1990) found that patients and their treating psychiatrists both agreed on the symptomatic benefits of major tranquillisers and their adverse social costs. Whilst patients did not want to suffer the latter (hence their 'non-compliance' at times), psychiatrists believed that the social benefits of tranquillisation were warranted. There is no disagreement between the two parties about costs and benefits but there is about the weighting given to each.

- Fourth, biological treatments are a restricted choice for service users, who want to maximise the treatments available or offered to them.
- Fifth, many users believe that biological treatments are more dangerous than talking treatments or they may even believe that the latter hold no dangers at all, despite evidence which points to their iatrogenic effects (see next chapter). This bias in user opinion may reflect the understandable range of distressing 'side-effects' medication has brought in the past to recipients, which are contrasted subjectively with the (reasonable) expectation of the alternative of drug free, respectful, benign conversations. The common term 'side effects' is put in speech marks because strictly they are disvalued *effects*.

The predictable, and sometimes very visible, adverse impact of drugs is a source of understandable concern for their recipients. Because psychotropic drugs act directly upon the central nervous system, they risk disturbing every, and any, part of CNS functioning (extending to others such as the endocrine and hepatic systems) as they are not magic bullets with specific target effects. They are more like a blunderbuss than a rifle. For this reason, some psychiatric critics of biological approaches, such as Breggin (1993), describe them as 'brain disabling'. Psychiatric drugs have been linked quite unambiguously to: sexual dysfunction; breast enlargement and lactation; menstrual disruption; liver dysfunction; Parkinsonism; tremor; dystonia; tardive dyskinesia; seizures; weight gain; bowel dysfunction; nausea; dry mouth; diuresis; cardio-toxicity; hypotension; memory disruption; dysphoria; irritability; akathisia; loss of motivation; panic attacks; and sedation. All of these adverse effects are fully acknowledged by those who are active advocates of drug treatments in psychiatry (e.g., Baldessarini 1999).

Many of these physiological and psychological effects in turn create social dysfunction or social dangers. For example, with sedation effects come an increased risk of traffic and other accidents. Psychiatric drugs have been directly linked to fractures and other injuries when prescribed to older people. By 1980 in Britain, one third of older people in residential homes were being given night sedation (Morgan and Gilleard 1981). By the late 1980s, the drug companies were spending over US $2 million just on advertising targeted at old-age physicians (Phillipson 1989).

The link between psychiatric drug use and raised levels of self-harm and harm to others has also been demonstrated. Some adverse drug effects are then treated with other drugs (an iatrogenically induced market). For example, TD cannot be countered, but other extra-pyramidal effects, such as stiffness and tremor, can be controlled by anticholinergic drugs. These may be given concurrently with neuroleptics. However, these drugs can produce their own adverse effects such as agitation. They can also be used for self-poisoning.

We noted earlier the increased use of psychiatric drugs with children in recent years, which raises specific questions about the potential long-term dangers imposed upon an immature neurological system. Also, some racial groups appear to be more sensitive to iatrogenic effects than others. For example, Jewish patients and those of African origin (which are overrepresented in groups diagnosed as psychotic) are more susceptible to agranulocytosis, an adverse risk in one of the newer anti-psychotics, clozapine (Fisher and Baigent 1996). Another group, which is particularly sensitive to the life threatening neuroleptic malignant syndrome, is asthmatic patients. These have significantly higher rates of iatrogenic death from neuroleptics than non-asthmatics (Joseph *et al.* 1996).

When all the above points are considered together, user opposition to biological treatments is highly intelligible. The extent to which lay knowledge and experiences are taken as valid and are able to permeate policy making at different levels is also likely to impact on a policy agenda which seeks to reverse social exclusion. An example here relates to what is included or excluded as gold standard 'evidence'. Notwithstanding the problems that may or may not be associated with the new generation of atypical anti-psychotic drugs, one of their potential advantages may be a reduction in side effects which in turn may have implications for social functioning and a reduction in stigma. (The latter, as we have seen in Chapter 4, are central to levels of social rejection for people living in ordinary communities).

Systematic reviews based to a large extent on the results produced by randomised controlled trials (RCTs) provide the accepted 'gold standard' evidence-base for medical practice. They hold considerable sway in the making of judgements[3] about whether the newer anti-psychotics (which are much more expensive) are to be made widely accessible and available via the NHS. A recent review excluded from consideration the inclusion of user views from a systematic review published in the *British Medical Journal*, which recommended the continued used of the old anti-psychotics as first-choice treatment (Geddes *et al.* 2000). The authors acknowledged the poor quality of the studies used as the basis of the review but continued to use as their main outcome measure professionally rated symptom rates and side effects. The failure to include user-defined outcomes was not mentioned as a weakness of the studies forming the basis of the review or indeed as a caveat to the recommendation about continued use of 'old' anti-psychotics. Prior *et al.* (2001) make the point, in response to the Geddes *et al.* review, that lay knowledge provides a difference in emphases which impacts on how the value of anti-psychotics should be evaluated:

> We urge clinicians to stop and think before accepting Geddes *et al.*'s results. It can be profoundly traumatic to be rendered rigid, trembling, unable to rest or obese by drug treatment and still coming to terms with the diagnosis, the stigma and the loss of hopes and expectations. (Prior, Clements and Rowett 2000)

The implications are that the inclusion of knowledge based on users' defined and personal experiences of taking anti-psychotics is likely to lead to different conclusions about their role in social exclusion and the quality of lives of psychiatric patients. Having provided a critical review of drug treatments, we will now discuss their wider context.

Putting biological treatments in context

The dominance of biological treatments in psychiatry is a function of three main drivers: medical knowledge; the pharmaceutical industry; and the social control role of mental health services. Because drugs are the staple medical response to mental health problems, we have focused on them above. However, lesser used treatments, such as ECT and psychosurgery, can still be found in the 'therapeutic armamentarium' of psychiatry. Like drugs, these tend to be given differentially. Poorer patients are more likely to receive ECT, as are women. Whilst adults receive ECT in the main, its use is not unknown in children.

Currently, there is a clear conflict between professional opinion about the utility of ECT and that offered by service users when surveyed (Royal College of Psychiatrists 1996). Basically, professionals argue that ECT is effective for severe depression and that it is linked to no long-term adverse effects. For psychiatrists, the question of the quality of ECT use is only about assessing the patient's suitability and auditing good practice when it is administered. ECT is discussed in the professional literature in these terms alone – its effectiveness at rescuing people from major depression is simply taken for granted. In contrast, users complain that it is a very frightening treatment and that it causes long-term problems of memory loss in its recipients. Professionals also argue that it is a treatment of last resort. However, we found in a survey of patients that nearly half of our sample, with a range of diagnoses, had received ECT (Rogers *et al.* 1993). We also found, however, that ECT produced the widest range of user opinion (with some arguing that it was an abomination which justified it being criminalised and others saying that it saved their lives).

Conclusion

The dominance of drug treatments has created a situation in mental health services in which a form of pseudo-democracy is to some degree imposed. Most patients get drugs, whether they want them are not. The great majority of patients with mental health problems are prescribed psychotropic drugs by primary care physicians or by psychiatrists (Rogers *et al.* 1993). The apparent lack of inequality in drug treatments, compared to talking treatments with their 'YAVIS' effect, is Fordist in nature (see p. 214). Ford famously told his customers that they could have their car in any colour provided that it was black. This imposed access to drugs has been linked with a number of features:

- Users resent the lack of choice in psychiatric treatment.
- Some groups (such as the National Schizophrenia Fellowship) campaign for greater access to drugs which might be restricted on grounds of cost, such as the newer anti-psychotics.
- Psychiatrists typically conflate the concept of 'treatment' with 'medication'. This can also be found in politicians establishing or reforming mental health policy and in ensuing debates in the mass media. For example, recurring debates about the use of enforced treatment orders in the community (CTOs) or concerns about 'treatment compliance' in discharged psychiatric patients focus singularly on the receipt of psychotropic drugs.
- Whether we examine the professional practice of psychiatrists about drugs or ECT (psychosurgery is more contested within the profession), the overall sense is one of complacency or denial, with a 'business-as-usual' response to criticism. For example, despite the well-established evidence about their dangers, mega-dosing and polypharmacy are still common-place in psychiatric practice. At other times, there are silences. For example, the dangers of akathisia associated with major tranquillisers were established clearly in the 1970s (Van Putten 1975). Despite this, in the subsequent twenty-five years no Royal College or any other psychiatric conference has been organised about it in the UK (Healy 2000). Another example is phased silence. Before the introduction of the newer atypical anti-psychotics, concerns about TD and akathisia were not conceded on a regular basis by professionals (Brown and Funk 1986). However, once the newer drugs were introduced, psychiatrists began to talk about the problems with the older drugs.
- The evasion of responsibility for the iatrogenic consequences of drug treatments from psychiatrists and the pharmaceutical industry has taken two forms. First, severity of illness has been used to warrant the use of imperfect drugs and justify the tolerance of clinical iatrogenesis (Finn *et al.* 1990). Second, 'side-effects' such as TD and akathisia have sometimes been attributed to the patient's illness, not their treatment – the ultimate form of victim blaming (Healy 2000; Van Putten 1975).

If we stand back from the competitive biological versus psychological treatment debate, what does the cost–benefit balance sheet
of drug treatments tell us? First, they do not cure but they do help
some people some of the time. All the drugs licensed for public consumption have been shown to be effective at creating symptomatic
relief compared to placebos in randomised controlled trials. In other
words, they are clinically effective, even if their cost-effectiveness is
contested.

Second, their benefits to recipients are confounded strongly
with adverse effects, with the latter impacting negatively upon
physiological, psychological and social functioning. Given the
widespread use of drugs, more controversial treatments (such as
ECT and psychosurgery) are actually relatively small beer because
their use is more restricted. Of all the treatments prescribed by
psychiatry in the last fifty years, tranquillisers (major and minor)
have created the largest iatrogenic toll because of the high rates of
their prescription.

Third, on the part of the psychiatric profession there has been
a reluctance to reflect on the costs and benefits of biologically
dominated practice (although a few dissenting members of the profession have stood out in this regard). Some competing professionals
have embraced the critical role more enthusiastically (for example,
Cohen, Fisher and Greenberg are psychologists cited earlier), which
is less surprising.

Fourth, and following from this point, what professionals say that
research tells us about biological treatments and what patients tell us
are different in many respects. This is not just about professionals
minimising adverse publicity about their capability in their role, it is
also about their utilising criteria of social regulation not just the
amelioration of distress. Put simply, if patients claim that they are
the new experts via experience, professionals remind us that their
expertise should remain pre-eminent and that they are the permanent 'guardian of the lunatic'.

Given the above point about biological treatments being Fordist,
as they commonly are used in a conveyer-belt manner in services,
with little or no consumer choice, it is understandable why people
with mental health problems, and their relatives, have recurrently
asked for alternatives. The weakest level of this demand was
mentioned in relation to the National Schizophrenia Fellowship
campaign to have greater access to the newer anti-psychotics. The

stronger version is the demand for more talking treatments and less biological treatments from the users' movement. For example, the founding charter of Survivors Speak Out in 1988 demanded 'free counselling for all'. In the light of this political demand, we turn in the next and final chapters to the question of talking treatments. Are they a worthy alternative to biological treatments?

9

Talking treatments: some are more equal than others

Introduction

Mental health work has often been caricatured as a form of talking treatment. The picture of the analyst with his (*sic*) patient reclining on a couch has been a recurring and emblematic image in North American and European culture. In this media-fuelled, popular imagination, psychiatry, psychology and psychoanalysis became synonymous. However, when we move from these imaginings to the more prosaic reality of NHS psychiatry a yawning gap is created.

Given the common expectation of mental health work, that it is about personal accounts being listened to respectfully for hour upon hour, people with mental health problems often get a rude awakening. Indeed, we have argued elsewhere (Rogers *et al.* 1993) that at least some of the disaffection expressed by psychiatric patients about the services they receive has been because of such failed expectations. Whilst 98 per cent of British psychiatric patients receive drug treatment, only around 60 per cent report receiving some form of psychological intervention, and some of this is obtained outside the NHS. Here, we deal with talking treatments from the perspective of inequalities. In particular, the following questions will be addressed:

- Are talking treatments determined by psychiatric diagnosis?
- Are talking treatments offered differentially according to socio-economic status?
- Are talking treatments racialised?
- Do talking treatments favour certain age groups and not others?
- Are talking treatments offered equally to men and women?

Having gathered some evidence in response to these questions, we will discuss the additive picture across all five. At the end of the chapter, we look at the question of therapeutic outcome in the light of debates about equality of access.

Different access to talking treatments is determined by psychiatric diagnosis

Conceptually, diagnosis is sometimes used as a means of defining suitability for talking treatments. For example, a psychotic patient, or one with a severe drink problem or personality problem, may be considered to be so incoherent or disorganised that a therapist may lack confidence in the client's capacity to honour the social contract about voluntary attendance at an agreed time and place. In the psychoanalytical tradition, as we note later, the formation of a transference relationship is of central importance *for the therapist* to make therapy possible. Psychotic patients are deemed, because of their weak ego functioning, to lack a capacity to form a transference or they are seen to have real direct personal needs rather than a need for learning via an interpretive method in therapy (Kernberg 1973).

A deeper professional accommodation has attended this reticence of psychotherapists to engage with people with psychotic problems. Essentially, a division of labour has emerged in the mental health industry, whereby biological psychiatrists have retained the dominant managerial responsibility for madness, with neurosis in all its forms (from general anxiety states and specific phobias to mild to moderate depression and obsessive-compulsive problems) being relinquished to medical and non-medical psychotherapists. Consequently, most of the literature about psychological therapies relates to this latter range of expressions of psychosocial misery.

Turning to empirical studies, early investigations of deterioration effects in therapy tended to confirm psychotherapeutic pessimism about patients with a diagnosis of psychosis or personality disorder (Lambert and Bergin 1994). These summary conclusions from Lambert and Bergin were pointedly about traditional one-to-one psychodynamic psychotherapy or humanistic group therapy (the encounter group tradition). However, some types of psychosocial intervention have been specifically designed for working with 'severe mental illness'. These include psycho-educational and problem-solving methods with patients and their families, behaviour therapy and cognitive therapy with individual clients. These methods have been shown to be effective at altering psychotic conduct as uni-therapies or in combination with anti-psychotic medication (Klerman *et al.* 1994). Also, some reviewers maintained (*contra* Lambert and Bergin 1994) that individual psychotherapy should be the 'treatment of choice' for psychotic patients on the grounds of its efficacy (Karon and VandenBos 1981).

However, the empirical demonstration of the effectiveness of tailored psychological methods for psychosis have not neatly transferred into mental health services. This is even true of methods ('psychosocial interventions') such as those developed by psychiatrists, which are not an ideological challenge to the illness model about diagnoses such as 'schizophrenia'. Thus, whilst a range of psychological methods have had a 'good press' in the research literature, service systems seem to resist their adoption. In contrast, as we have seen in the previous chapter, drug treatments have a predictable and often monopoly status in service responses to psychosis.

Talking treatments are offered differentially according to socio-economic status

A series of large-scale studies have demonstrated quite clearly that income, employment status and years in education are correlated with the receipt of psychotherapy, when people present with mental health problems (Hollingshead and Redlich 1958; Kadushin 1969; Lubin *et al.* 1973; Olfson and Pincus 1999; Ryan 1969; Weber *et al.* 1985). Not only are poorer clients with the same symptom profiles as richer equivalents less likely to be offered psychotherapy, they are more likely to be prescribed drugs and ECT. The sources of this class gradient in treatment allocation include the access richer clients have to therapist choice in the private sector, referrer bias and discrimination at the point of assessment by therapists.

Not only are poorer patients less likely to be offered talking treatments, they are also more likely to fail to attend the initial appointment offered and also to drop out from treatment earlier than richer patients (Berrigan and Garfield 1981; Pilkonis *et al.* 1984). The Berrigan and Garfield study demonstrated a clear linear relationship between social class and continuation in therapy. This picture was also apparent in the dropout pattern of those attending

NHS outpatient treatment with clinical psychologists (Weighill *et al.* 1983). This suggests that fee payment is not an influence in dropout but that the latter reflects a lack of confidence by poorer clients in the rationale or utility of psychological treatments.

Are talking treatments racialised?

Later, we discuss the racial underpinnings of psychotherapeutic models, but here we address the empirical issue of racial differences in treatment allocation. Generally, the evidence suggests that black patients are less likely to be offered psychotherapy in North America and Europe. As with social class, a racial effect is apparent in relation to dropout from therapy, at least according to early studies. Non-white clients were shown to drop out earlier than whites (Salzman *et al.* 1970; Yamamoto *et al.* 1968). However, Garfield (1994) noted that later studies showed mixed results – some continued to show the earlier picture, others showed no racial differences in dropout. Garfield speculates that a cultural shift in the mental health workforce about race (in the USA) may account for this later convergence. He also makes the important methodological point that many of the studies of black and ethnic minority clients have not partialed out social class factors and so firm conclusions about any racial effect, if found, cannot be made.

In those studies which have been more focused on racial and cultural variables, ethnic and linguistic matching between therapists and clients seem to predict better outcomes and fewer dropouts (Sue *et al.* 1991). In Britain, several studies have shown that black patients are more likely to receive physical treatments than psychological treatments. This point extends to racial differences in levels of coercion (see Chapter 3). Thus, the evidence on race is less clear-cut than on social class, although decision-making biases against black and ethnic minorities can be seen in relation to psychotherapy.

Do talking treatments favour some age groups and not others?

Generally mental health services throughout the life-span show a decreasing tendency to offer psychological treatments (Olfson and Pincus 1999). Although child and adolescent mental health services receive less political attention and resourcing than those for people of working age, their internal treatment priorities tend to be more psychological than somatic. There is a general consensus across the mental health professions that they are dealing with an immature client group which *ipso facto* is experiencing concurrent biological, psychological and social developmental changes. The immediate relationship between family and school milieu and the behaviour of young people is more clear-cut than the behavioural linkages which might exist between adults with mental health problems and their living context.

Mental health work with younger people thus has an opportunity to intervene with and harness a change process which is normal by dint of age. Also, as we noted in the previous chapter, because of the immaturity of the central nervous system, many child psychiatrists, out of caution, are prone to use less medication than their colleagues working with adult patients. These factors together produce a more psychologically oriented ethos in child and adolescent mental health services, with individual and family therapy being commonplace. Moreover, the differing conceptual underpinnings of mental health work all have a developmental motif. Social learning, cognitive development, psycho-sexual development, classical and operant conditioning, etc. are components of psychological models in general. Consequently they have an immediate temporal relevance when working with children.

Notwithstanding the points made outside this section about class, race and gender, adults of working age with mental health problems are less likely to receive psychological interventions than are children but more likely to do so than those beyond retirement age. Older people tend to be offered less psychotherapy but tend to drop out less frequently than younger clients. Although Jung and Erikson placed an emphasis upon the integrative function and developmental challenges of ageing, other depth psychologists have avoided older clients. Freud argued that age brings psychological rigidity and so older people are less open to interpretive influence compared to younger people. He basically argued that the older we get, the less treatable we become.

Are talking treatments offered equally to men and women?

The answer to this is definitely in the negative. Women are in receipt of more psychiatric interventions than men, including talking treatments. The reasons for this include sex differences in help-seeking (women have more primary health care consultations than men) and sex differences in presenting problems. For example, sex differences in prevalence rates of psychiatric morbidity virtually disappear if personality disorder and drug and alcohol problems are included in epidemiological data. Women are twice as likely as men to present with problems which fall within the traditional target remit of the talking treatments (depression and anxiety-based problems). Also, the inflated prevalence rates of mental disorder typically quoted about women are partially accounted for by their living longer. This provides more time for women to incur functional problems such as depression, not just dementia.

The mental health service profile is associated with a gradient of treatments – secondary services are linked to more enforced and biological treatments, whereas primary care consultations are all voluntary and they mix drug and psychological treatments. Because many more patients are diagnosed and treated for mental health problems in primary care than secondary care (see Chapter 4), this raises both the incidence and prevalence of female diagnosis because of their higher rate of voluntary, community-based consultations. It also makes it more likely for women than men to receive both drug *and* psychological treatment. Men now predominate in inpatient settings where drug treatments are ubiquitous but psychological treatments are not common.

The political responsibility of therapists for unequal access

Having pulled together evidence from a variety of sources that talking treatments are not delivered equitably in our society, what conclusions can we draw? Clearly each question addressed above indicates not one but several aspects of inequality which permeate professional practice. The latter entails therapists paying heed to biographical data and, through that process, attempting to enable or negotiate mental health gain with their clients. Whilst people are rarely explicitly excluded categorically on *a priori* grounds from talking treatments, in practice the lives of some rather than others are more likely to be deemed worthy of a biographical dialogue. Put differently, the eventual client group for psychotherapists is more likely to be: neurotic rather than psychotic; richer rather than poorer; white rather than black; young rather than old; and female not male. In the psychotherapy literature, this is known as the YAVIS phenomenon (the therapy client being stereotypically young, attractive, verbal, intelligent and social).

It would be tempting, given this set of demonstrable biases, to attribute the broad picture of inequality of access to a conscious or unconscious preference of therapists to work with some types of people and not others. Indeed, some psychodynamic commentators on the relative exclusion of older people have argued that age discrimination simply reflects the aggregate effect of negative counter-transference (or, in non-psychoanalytical language, the cumulative ageist prejudices of therapists) (Hildebrand 1982). This notion of the outcome of differential treatment of clients reflecting a process of preferential treatment by therapists may have some validity, but it is also reductive and unifactorial as a hypothesis. In its favour, we can point to a number of sources of evidence but we also need to rehearse cautions and counterclaims as well. Freud treated neurotics and, in his tradition, therapists argue that psychotic patients cannot form a transference relationship and so are untreatable. On the other hand, a number of psychological therapists have deliberately set out to work with psychotic clients and so the latter have not been ruled out of consideration *en masse* by all therapists.

With regards to socio-economic status, those clients who can pay can shop around for therapists, many of whom earn their living wholly or partially in private practice. Given this cash nexus as a defining feature of much of the psychotherapy industry, the richer client will be favoured. At the same time, many psychological therapists are committed to publicly funded organisations such as the NHS and refuse to practice privately exclusively, or may do so only on a part-time basis. Freud was ambivalent about the fee, arguing sometimes that it was a vital point of interpretation in the relationship and at other times that analysts should treat some patients free. His followers continued to reflect this ambivalence after his death (Power and Pilgrim 1990). Thus, whilst many therapists may be biased towards private practice, maybe even seeing it as a virtue not a form of discrimination, this generalisation by no means holds true for all practitioners. Using economic relationships as a defining feature of political values, psychotherapists often can be accused of elitism but many are unjust targets for this accusation.

With regards to race, the dominant models of Western psychotherapy are certainly open to inspection but the racial interests they may reflect are neither uniform nor straightforward. Although many models of talking treatments exist, three approaches predominate (cognitive, humanistic and psychodynamic). The two seminal proponents of cognitive therapy (Beck and Ellis) are from the USA but the theoretical roots of cognitive therapy lie in Russian behaviourism and British associationism (Pilgrim and Treacher 1992) and, to some degree, the reaction of Ellis against his original psychoanalytical training. (Beck's approach is much more pragmatic than theory-driven.) The seemingly paradoxical notion of 'cognitive-behaviour therapy' represents a coalescing of empirical findings from physiological experiments, philosophical models derived from introspection and a rationalistic rejection of depth psychology. The point of importance here is that cognitive therapy was derived from a geographical space in one part of the Northern hemisphere (mainly Europe). As a result, the cultural features of this geographical source are immanent in cognitive therapy. Other cultural resonances (for example Asian, South American or African) are missing, although some cognitive therapists have recently developed techniques which draw explicitly on older Eastern ways, such as Zen Buddhism (Linehan 1995).

In the humanistic tradition from North America, the models set out by Rogers, Kelly and Maslow are deeply personalistic and place a great deal of emphasis upon individual agency, not social structure. This may well reflect a recycling of white American cultural assumptions about free will, a respect for the autonomous individual, and a democratic assumption (or collective delusion) that 'anyone can become President'. These assumptions were fed by two different political dynamics. On the one hand, the civil libertarian reaction against slavery installed individual freedom as a cornerstone of American political values. On the other hand, the thrill and virtue of breaking any frontier was linked to the destruction of, not respect for, the rights of others (capturing land and killing indigenous American 'Indians' and razing Vietnamese villages).

Beneath this American cultural dimension about human potential is the historically imported Protestantism from one aspect of a non-conformist, anti-clerical, European Christianity, with its emphasis on personal responsibility. However, whilst these resonances are visible (for those who look for them), their processing in a liberal secular mode during the twentieth century also reshaped their emphasis in an uneven way. Although the human potential movement took the notion of individual agency to absurd proportions, others such as Kelly placed a particular emphasis upon how the social context shapes a person's way of construing their world (Kelly 1955). As for Rogers, he pursued a genuine desire for a peaceful just world in many of his later projects.

Turning to psychoanalysis, the Freudian project was one of a secular Jewish leader surrounded by those of a similar background with only one exceptional Gentile (Jung) temporarily in its midst. Whilst the Nazis burned psychoanalytical texts, Jung's theories were highly compatible with theories of Aryan supremacy and he was offered a protected status in Germanic psychiatry during the Second World War (Masson 1988; Noll 1996). If Jung and his views are excluded, psychoanalysis can be seen (like American humanism noted above) as a reflection of prior cultural assumptions–largely ones of Judaistic explorations of inner life and the tensions of living in a moral order. This is a cultural world of recurring moral concerns in which conscience struggles with desire and the intellect plays with unreason.

Thus, American humanism and psychoanalysis, the predominant forces which have shaped pure and derived styles of talking treatment, were undoubtedly racial (i.e., European) in their origins but by no stretch of the imagination can they be described as *racist* in their assumptions or aspirations, provided that Carl Jung is left out of the picture. Indeed, by and large, the opposite seems to be true of practising therapists who, driven by their therapeutic ideology, are highly respectful of the uniqueness of individual experience. Moreover, compared to the eugenic emphasis in the theoretical underpinnings of biological psychiatry which we dealt with in the previous chapter, psychotherapists have a relatively honourable history in relation to their implicit political values, which tend to be tolerant and liberal or leftist in their personal political value systems (Samuels 1998).

Nonetheless, in a contemporary multicultural society the European origins of psychotherapy, all of which have been refracted through the prism of modern North American secular culture, are not suited to all-comers. Questions of agency and individualism are reflected on differently by secular Western psychotherapists, be they cognitive, humanistic or psychodynamic in orientation, than by, say, a Hindu or a Muslim with no training in mental health work. For example, traditional Asian values about social rather than personal priorities, shame, filial piety, fatalism and inconspicuousness are out of sync with white American individualism and its mirroring in humanistic psychology and ego psychology (Kitano and Maki 1996).

When we turn to gender, a seeming paradox emerges. An oppressed status defined by class (low), age (old) or diagnosis (psychosis) consistently predicts a raised probability of exclusion from psychotherapy. Consequently, the post-feminist consensus that women are oppressed more than, and generally by, men might lead us to expect the relative exclusion of women from talking treatments. But this is not the case. The dominant discourse about gender and therapy has been dominated by the confluence of feminist *and* psychoanalytical ideologies during the 1970s in Europe and North America (Chodorow 1978; Eichenbaum and Orbach 1983; Lawrence and Maguire 1997; Mitchell 1974), although at times feminist opposition to this marriage of convenience has been evident (e.g., Tennov 1976). This hybrid of feminism and psychoanalysis has produced a skewing of the discussion about gender and psychotherapy. This has created a silence about the relative absence of men from voluntary psychological treatments and about male issues in therapy. Although women are treated for mental health problems more often than men, this discrepancy is accounted for, overwhelmingly, by voluntary encounters with professionals, especially in primary care. By contrast, the mental health industry is more likely to be imposed coercively upon men. Thus, men suffer a double structural disadvantage compared to women: they are poorer help-seekers; and they are treated coercively more often. These two factors create the conditions in which men are excluded from talking treatments more often than women.

Another consequence of the feminism–psychoanalysis conflation has been that psychotherapy for *women* has been conflated non-problematically with psychodynamic therapy. For example, the misleadingly titled edited collection by Lawrence and Maguire (*ibid.*) is *Psychotherapy with Women: Feminist Perspectives*. In fact, the book is only written from a psychodynamic perspective. This perspective limits the capacity of students of gender, psychotherapy and mental health to reflect critically outside, and about, psychoanalysis as the latter is accepted as *the* way of understanding the relationship between inner and outer life. Even texts which concede a more pluralistic set of possibilities about women and therapy still rely predominantly on psychodynamic ideas (e.g., Walker 1990). Recently, the psychodynamic discourse about gender has been disrupted by postmodern critiques which bring men into the equation as possessors, not just creators, of mental health problems (Law 1999) and explore power and gender in the therapeutic relationship in a range of ways (Swan 1999).

Thus, women therapists cannot be accused of being gender-blind in their writings, but there has been a recent tendency mainly to attend to only half of the population (as 'gender' or 'sex' have come overwhelmingly to mean 'women') or to consider men as only causes not possessors of mental health problems (e.g., Ussher and Nicolson 1992). Moreover, the predominant alliance with depth psychology has incorporated the weaknesses of the latter as a form of *social* science. For example, the problems of Freud's misogyny, his betrayal of patients who were incest victims, the psychological reductionism of his whole subsequent tradition or Jung's racism are ignored, dealt with superficially, or rationalised by the feminist therapists cited above (Pilgrim 1997).

External influences on differential access

Having noted the grounds for suspecting the discriminatory motives of psychotherapists and then rehearsed some counter-arguments, the evidence gathered earlier in the chapter remains. If therapists themselves are not wholly responsible for inequalities in access to talking treatments, which other factors do we need to consider? Broadly, three points could be made to bring in other interests outside the culture of the talking treatments that shape its character.

First, there is the general *therapeutic pessimism surrounding psychosis and personality disorder* and the political imperative to control madness and dangerous conduct. It is clear from Chapters 3 and 4 that the mental health industry is not solely in the business of reducing distress in a context of voluntary service contact. A good chunk of its work entails the management of risky behaviour and the suppression of forms of deviance that are a threat to the moral and economic workings of society. In this light, decisions are made about patients that are at times about controlling their risk and managing their chronic social disability.

These more dominant themes in mental health work with psychotic patients displace other considerations (such as the exploration of inner life). Indeed, until recently, when some cognitive therapists have sought to engage with deluded or hallucinating patients, the norm in mental health work has been deliberately to eschew any meaningful dialogue with madness. This, amongst other reasons, is why the British and French 'anti-psychiatrists' were considered beyond the pale by orthodox mental health workers in the 1970s. Therapists such as R.D. Laing, who was both a psychiatrist and psychoanalyst, attempted to render madness intelligible via conversations with psychotic patients. This project contrasts starkly with the pessimism created by the view since Kraepelin that madness is a biologically fixed, deteriorating condition – the main assumption behind the social drift theory in psychiatry (see Chapter 1) and the unremitting emphasis upon genetic and other forms of biological research about psychosis (Bentall *et al.* 1988).

When interventions are involuntary, as they episodically are with psychotic patients, and sometimes are semi-permanently with 'personality disordered' offenders, then a basic tenet of talking treatments is violated, that of voluntarism. Psychological therapies rely in part on the voluntary motivation of their clients in order for the latter to set and pursue meaningful goals in their life. Thus, it is not only the willingness of biological psychiatrists to acquire a predominant authority about madness, it is also the reticence of most psychological therapists to become involved in this area. The upshot of these dynamics of the social management of madness is that the psychotic is typically deemed insufficiently worthy of personal respect to warrant a sustained biographical dialogue. As a consequence, their treatment is typically physical.

Second, there is the *centrality of language*. Talking treatments, *ipso facto*, rely predominantly upon talk. For this reason, they can only maximise their potential if the therapist and client start from a shared linguistic culture. In its grossest sense it is obvious, for example, that psychoanalysis is impossible when the analyst and their analysand speak different languages. But there are gradations of this point. For example, in New York, an unemployed Latino will understand their world differently from a comfortable Jewish psychoanalyst. Both will be able to communicate well enough with some shared version of North American English, but there will also be much of the linguistic worlds of each of the two parties which is alien to the other. The words they use reflect, and partially constitute, their different inhabited worlds. The nuances and inflections of meaning brought by the patient to an account of their life would be missed episodically and maybe sometimes crucially by the therapist in the relationship.

The class basis of discrepant linguistic frameworks was described by Bernstein in his notions of restricted and elaborated codes. This approach focused upon the educational and familial linguistic differences between working-class and middle-class people. As well as differences in learning, cultures lead to poorer educated children developing a more restricted use of language, their restricted code is considered to be more action-oriented and less reflective than, for example, the world inhabited by psychotherapists.

Third, there are a set of *structural factors* which determine higher rates of distress and madness in oppressed groups. These are the groups which are disproportionately represented in psychiatric populations. The cumulative stressor effects of material deprivation, racism, ageism and sexism propel some groups into help-seeking for distress (e.g., white / women) more than others (e.g., black / men). The latter groups may predominantly express their psychological abnormality through disruptive acting out: madness, substance abuse and violence (see Chapter 6). As a consequence, the response of services will be more about risk management than psychotherapy in these circumstances.

The outcome debate and inequalities

Finally, in this chapter we need to note the controversy about the effectiveness of talking treatments. Its relevance for our purposes is political – differential access has one meaning if talking treatments are effective and another if they are not. In the former case, higher rates of exclusion from therapy for some social groups would represent discriminatory service provision. If, by contrast, talking treatments were ineffective, this concern would be meaningless, at least at the level of a government health policy aspiring to create equality of access to effective treatments.

At the individual level, those in excluded groups may still experience oppression in relationship to being debarred from ineffective or unproven treatments. For example, the ability of richer neurotic people to buy private healing interventions, some of which may be of unproven efficacy, is part of their enjoyment of their cultural capital and their material privilege. Such an enjoyment would be denied to a poorer psychotic person. It is noteworthy in this regard that the mental health service users' movement has predominantly attacked the mode of therapy imposed most often by professionals (physical treatments) and demanded free access to talking treatments. Radical critics of psychotherapy are of the view that patients are misguided in this demand (Masson 1988).

Thus, although we cannot dwell at length on the complex arguments about the effectiveness of talking treatments, some summary points need to be made because effectiveness has become a political, not just a scientific, question.

(1) Efficacy studies

Those evaluating the worth of talking treatments have still not resolved the relative importance of efficacy compared to effectiveness. Efficacy is a pure version of outcome research which takes a selected group of patients with defined characteristics. A protocol-driven intervention ('treatment fidelity') is given to this group and not to another (control) group. Outcomes are evaluated by people who do not know how patients were assigned. When studying drug treatments, complete randomisation of patients to treatment and control groups can be ensured, as can the blindness of the therapist (who gives out dummy placebo tablets to half of his or her sample). As neither the therapist nor the patient are aware of which group the latter is in, drug efficacy trials are thus 'double-blind'. These ideal conditions of randomised controlled trials cannot be achieved with talking treatments, as both therapist and client know when a therapy is or is not being given. Nonetheless, intention to treat (waiting list) controls can be used and evaluated independently to see whether the passage of time brings with it changes compared to similar patients who are given therapy in the same time frame.

(2) Effectiveness studies

These quasi-experimental efficacy studies can be contrasted with a newer generation of *in situ* studies of effectiveness in services (Miller and Magruder 1999). In the latter regard, outcome measures are used (still with blind independent raters) on populations who are less selected and who receive therapy from practitioners who may not be protocol driven.

With this methodological point in mind, effectiveness studies have generated more optimistic (positive) findings than have efficacy studies, although both indicate that psychological therapies are effective when compared to no treatment.

(3) Consistency and reliability of approach

Three groups of patients are identified within this overall positive conclusion about outcome. There are those who improve significantly as a result of therapy. There are those who remain the same. A third group actually *deteriorate* when given therapy. Consequently, a therapist or their employing service cannot say with certainty in advance that a therapy offered will improve a specific mental health problem experienced by a particular client.

Reasons offered for the lack of improvement in the second and third groups relate to three factors. First, incompetent therapists may be operating – these are not actively harmful, at least by intent, but they may fail to adhere to the model they claim to use consistently – they do not offer treatment fidelity. There is some evidence that *consistency of approach* is positively correlated with good outcome. Second, therapists may aggravate or fail to improve a mental health problem because they do not offer a benign supportive, empathic and honest stance in the relationship. There is much evidence that a positive relationship is a predictor of good outcome. Indeed, this evidence about a *positive working relationship* indicates that this feature is independent of, and more important than, the technicalities of the espoused model favoured by particular therapists. Third, some therapists exploit their clients for their own sexual or emotional ends. Thus, *abusive therapists* create additional traumatic problems for some clients. If these factors have been identified accurately in the literature on deterioration effects, then this suggests that the effectiveness of therapy in practice is functioning below its full potential. Put differently, much stronger evidence of effectiveness would be generated if all therapists could be guaranteed to operate in a consistent, benign and non-exploitative way.

(4) Therapist–client relationship

This therapist-factor approach to outcome has been augmented by a relevant body of literature on the *therapist–client relationship* and its link to outcome. That is, in addition to the above point about a positive therapist stance, client variables are also considered. This poses questions about which therapy or therapists work best with which clients to generate good outcomes. This is where the outcome literature connects in particular with the contents of this chapter, as it brings into play questions of therapist–client compatibility and synergy. Say, for argument, a mental health service contains a predominance of positive, competent, non-abusive psychological therapists; if a client is only offered one model of therapy, then a good outcome would still only be ensured if the model is meaningful to the client. If the acceptability of the approach is not checked and fully negotiated by the referrer (not just the therapist), then dissatisfied or distrustful clients will simply drop out early or even fail to attend the first appointment offered. As we noted earlier, this is exactly what happens disproportionately with lower-class and black clients in relation to talking treatments. This issue of selectivity is made explicit by some forms of therapy. For example, in NHS settings clients are assessed for their suitability for psychodynamic psychotherapy. It is not uncommon, following such assessments, for therapists to reject the client with a note to the referrer emphasising why the client is unsuitable for treatment. (They may be deemed by the assessing therapist to be insufficiently psychologically minded or they may be judged to be incapable of forming and using the therapeutic transference.) Other models of therapy are less explicit about this selectivity but implicitly concede good and bad bets. For example, the literature on cognitive-behaviour therapy expects rapid and good outcomes for clients with some presenting symptoms but not others.

Thus, by examining the literature on outcome we are once more back into political territory. This is not narrowly a scientific question because, apart from the broad health policy issue about equity of access to effective treatments, other notions of power are highlighted. For example, the professional discretion to offer this or that treatment is evident. In a locality, this may leave a client who cannot pay in a position of 'take it or leave it' from services, whereas the latter will contain therapists who will always have other clients waiting to be seen as demand exceeds supply in publicly funded therapy systems. In the private (or euphemistically self-styled 'independent') sector, even though the client is paying for a service, the therapist still determines the mode of therapy on offer. The private client may be able to shop around but they cannot negotiate how each therapist they consider should practise their role. Also, the extent of professional power in talking treatments is evident in the studies – clients are at the mercy of their therapist. The latter, whether employed in the public sector or operating privately, may be positive, competent and non-abusive; on the other hand they may not be.

Because of the vulnerability of clients to therapist-induced deterioration, some critics of psychotherapy have selectively attended to this danger and argued that we would all be wise to eschew psychotherapy (Masson 1988). Also, some feminist critics have complained that the normative emphasis in therapeutic models will ultimately disempower, not empower, women (Kitzinger 1993). The literature on therapist sexual abuse generally points to abusive therapists being middle-aged and male and their victims young and female (although a minority of studies show now sex differences) (Pilgrim and Guinan 1999). Thus, the arguments and evidence about abuse and normative effects throw the oppressive potential of the talking treatments into sharp relief.

The empirical ambiguity in the outcome literature – talking treatments are effective overall but some clients may not be helped or may even be harmed – does pose a tantalising political question about access to the talking treatments. Should those who tend to be relatively excluded (male, black, poorer, psychotic and older people) complain or rejoice? Professional dominance over clients is palpable in the talking treatments which have been linked, overoptimistically by some disaffected psychiatric patients, to a safe, democratic, empowering alternative to the biological psychiatry we explored in the previous two chapters.

Psychiatric treatments and inequalities

Despite user disaffection with somatic treatments, the unwary preference for talking treatments and the resistance of professionals to change in their working preferences, all parties are still trapped in a discourse of treatment and cure. Both drugs and psychotherapy are forms of psychiatric *treatment*. Sometimes psychotherapy is actually called the 'talking cure'. Psychotherapists as well as biological psychiatrists use a language of pathology. Both talk of 'resistance' to treatment residing in the patient or 'the treatment of choice' for this or that condition, or a patient's 'suitability for treatment'. Both types of professional therapist have 'patients' (indeed, in psychoanalytical therapy this preferred term is used proudly and reliably, especially by non-medical therapists).

What underlies this discourse is the assumption of both professionals and their clients that with enough effort, currently in relation to individual cases and ultimately in relation to whole classes of patients, there will be a proven technical fix for misery and madness. The incremental research programme of randomised controlled trials examining this or that physical or psychological treatment targeted on patients fulfilling this or that set of DSM criteria reinforces this way of thinking about the societal response to mental health problems. In other words, the latter have retained a common clinical focus in debates about equality. This can be contrasted, for example, with the ways in which the disability movement has taken its stance to medicalised social policy (Oliver 1990). Here, Perkins, a clinical psychologist with a diagnosis of manic-depression, comments:

> For me the problem lies in our continued insistence in seeing madness in purely 'health' terms. Mental health legislation focuses on which treatments and services should be available and whether we should be forced to comply with them. The mental health world argues about which is better, physical treatments or talking therapies or complimentary therapies. I really don't mind – the domain is the same – one of treatment and cure. The wider disability movement did not reject medicalisation in favour of a nicer therapeutic approach. They rejected it in favour of rights – to employment, to be educated, to travel, to vote, to stand as a politician ... But still the mental health world puts most of its energies into debating which treatments and services people should have – rather than the rights that could transform our lives so much more profoundly.

This critical point about people with mental health problems having their identity and life chances defined by acquired or imposed professional therapy can help to reframe our agenda about mental health and equality. This shift of focus involves testing the limits, not of (equal access to) medicine, but of equality of citizenship. The stigma and invalidation of a diagnosis and the iatrogenic impact of treatment have been a significant part of the focus of user opposition to psychiatry. Thus, the term 'survivor' is often used in relation to 'surviving' the oppression of the psychiatric system. And yet, this language of critical opposition misleadingly maintains a narrow clinical focus because people with mental health problems have survived in a much broader sense. They have also survived their primary psychological impairments and rejection by civil society.

If psychiatry did not exist, would the conduct associated with madness, fear and misery be tolerated and valued by others more than in the past? Historical studies of madness give no indication that it was routinely acceptable in societies prior to its medicalisation (Rosen 1978). More recent studies of societies without psychiatric services still indicate that madness brings with it rejection and stereotyping (Westermeyer and Kroll 1978). Thus, patient opposition to their treatment is understandable, but it is also part of the problem, not the solution, as far as demystifying the relationship between madness and society is concerned.

Currently, biological treatments are one component of the biodeterminist ideology. Apart from clinical iatrogenesis, biodeterministic psychiatric knowledge generates social and cultural iatrogenesis (Illich 1977). Biological treatment is like junk mail – everybody gets it, whether or not it is requested, some find it useful and the lives of others are diminished by it. But whilst it remains the dominant response from professionals, it also limits our horizons. It traps professional and lay participants alike in a somatic discourse in which the patient's body is spotlighted so intensively, that the psychosocial relations which create, maintain or amplify mental health problems are cast into a dark shadow. In this spotlight, need is defined only as the need for psychiatric treatment. The plea of Perkins above is about illuminating and playing upon a wider stage.

If psychiatry were abolished, or its political prominence substantially eroded, new challenges would be exposed. How would those with mental health problems be treated (in its generic sense) by all parties in society? What would be the limits of achievable citizenship for those people who were (or had been) crazy or so profoundly anxious or miserable that their domestic and employment roles had been lost or rendered significantly inefficient? These questions point up an implicit social contract about entitlement to citizenship which can be traced back to antiquity. Traditionally, madness has been placed or has placed itself (depending on one's view of intentionality and human agency) outside the social contract. As a consequence, the non-mad, with little guilt but with much fear, have kept their distance, often physically but always psychologically, from the mad (Jodelet 1991). That breakdown of communication has been challenged in recent years by dissenting professionals and the users' movement.

And this is where professionals may still be a relevant force for change, rather than simply being self-interested when evading criticism of their work and seeking to retain the powers of paternalism associated with their therapeutic role. The historical evidence does not bode well for people with mental health problems being treated equally in society. This pessimistic conclusion can only be undermined if, now and in the future, people with mental health problems and dissenting professionals form a campaigning alliance about citizenship.

10

Conclusions

Introduction

In the book's introduction, we advocated a critical realist paradigm in order to illuminate the topic of mental health and inequality (Bhaskar 1998). This necessitates the need to look beyond the details of the findings of individual empirical research projects and the adoption of a critical perspective, which unpicks professional interests, exposes the societal role of professional practice and draws into the frame of analysis knowledge-claims about services, not just professionally preferred ones, about patients. Additionally, a requirement of pursuing this goal is to move beyond the empiricism of individual studies in order to provide a broader view of the possible linkages implicated in the creation and perpetuation of the social disadvantage associated with mental health problems.

By looking across a range of empirical studies and analysis about mental health, it is clear that the two seemingly separate worlds of the 'causes' and constructs of social and behavioural problems and their 'treatment' and 'management' are permeable domains. By considering the two together, new types of explanations about mental health inequalities are made more possible. Thus, having raised questions about the limits of psychiatric epidemiology in the first two chapters of the book, we began to explore what had not happened (for example, the lack of a dialogue between the literature on service contact and that on epidemiology). We also sought to identify the social forces shaping the pre-empirical constructs which characterise social psychiatric research and to move from a scrutiny of static relationships (between socio-economic status and mental health) to dynamic relationships in open social systems. These dynamic relationships include, as we explored in Chapter 2, the interplay between poor places, poor people, their experience of poverty and the identity this creates.

Over many years, psychiatric epidemiology established that higher prevalence rates for a range of mental health problems were to be found amongst those in the lowest social classes. It also explored a range of factors that can account for this. Subsequently, both gender and race were identified as key variables linking social status and position to rates of mental health problems. However, as we argued in Chapter 1, over its changing form during the last 150 years, psychiatric knowledge has sometimes exposed social inequalities and sometimes acted in the interest of conservative social forces. At times, it may even have acted to obscure social causes and contributed to the maintenance of social divisions.

The mental health and public health reform movements of the nineteenth century were imbued with a moral and reforming thrust aimed at the poor. Victorian psychiatric epidemiology was bound up with a broad eugenic social policy of segregating an assumed 'tainted' gene pool. During the twentieth century, for a while, psychiatric epidemiology was associated with a more enlightened view of the needs of those with mental health problems. A social administrative phase, in which hospital samples and clinical diagnoses were used to describe the patterning of mental illness, was replaced with a post-Second World War generation of epidemiological studies, which demonstrated the influence of poverty and deprivation and pointed to social isolation, the influence of social factors that spanned the life-course and the experience of early infancy as likely aetiological factors. This generation of research on inequalities in mental health began to follow those evident in mainstream public health, with a focus on environmental conditions and the quality of interpersonal relationships in different parts of society.

Subsequently, a range of studies identified the relationship between mental health and social class. They demonstrated a consistent social patterning of mental disorders in which the rates of mental health problems were more prevalent amongst those in the 'lower' classes, although the link for 'common mental health problems' (anxiety and depression) appeared to be less consistent than the finding for schizophrenia. This approach has had utility too, when providing evidence for an inverse relationship between lower social position and mental health. Similar evidence is now available about race and gender, although this is more ambiguous.

However, the third generation of psychiatric epidemiology shifted its focus from society (and, thus, potentially social injustice) to its own internal workings. Methodological preoccupations and its standing within medical science came to dominate the field. Thus, when 'progressing' over time, psychiatric epidemiology became more professionally introverted and conservative in its norms. The great bulk of its products since the Second World War can be read without any sense that the mental health industry has endured recurring crises of credibility, fuelled first by academic and clinical dissent ('anti-psychiatry') and then by the growth of an oppositional new social movement (the users' movement). These voices of criticism attacked both the knowledge-base of psychiatry and the repressive role of clinicians. Social psychiatrists predominantly carried on regardless or, if engaging with the debates, played a bullish reactionary role on behalf of 'scientific medicine' and the profession of psychiatry. As an indication of an unresolved problematic, the profession's woes have continued with the emergence of 'critical psychiatry'; the postmodern equivalent of the 'anti-psychiatry' in the humanistic, libertarian, counter-culture of the 1960s.

The shortcomings of psychiatric epidemiology

Despite bringing poverty and social disadvantage into the frame of analysis, social psychiatry has been encumbered by a number of shortcomings arising from its reliance on its own shifting brand of epidemiology. We explored these in the early chapters of the book. As we argued in Chapter 1, despite the introduction of a more sophisticated psychosocial perspective, in many respects advances beyond the theoretical dichotomisation of, or compromises surrounding, the positions of social causation and social drift have been slow to emerge. The way in which the influences on mental health problems have been conceptualised remained limited, and, to a large extent, individualised. This, in turn, has limited the development of specific policy measures to address inequalities.

Conventional epidemiological studies have tended to pursue methodological credibility by seeking to improve the reliability and validity of the key variables of mental illness (for example, by adopting more stringent DSM criteria). Whilst this may have increased the scientific credentials of psychiatric epidemiology and boosted the self-confidence of social psychiatry as a medical speciality, a price has been paid. The newer epidemiology has become disconnected from a clear social environmentalist perspective and an individualistic model of psychopathology, divorced from wider social and material influences, has been reinforced. Consequently, certain possibilities have been undermined or lost, such as a focus on the relationship between social disadvantage and mental distress or the production of ameliorative solutions or recommendations. The redirection of the research endeavour within psychiatric epidemiology also had a political significance within the profession of psychiatry.

Biological psychiatry has been criticised recurrently as a perpetuator of inequalities, which might imply that such a charge is not applicable to social psychiatry. However, a version of the latter, increasingly self-conscious about its medical respectability, has tended to claim agnosticism about aetiology (in accordance with the epistemological position of DSM) or conceded the likelihood of biological suscepti-bility. In doing so, arguably, it has failed clearly and consistently to distance itself from bioreductionism in the mainstream of the psychiatric profession. A 'stress-vulnerability' position in social psychiatry is not incompatible with a biomedical model.

The link between mental health inequalities and service provision and professional knowledge

A further problem in existing approaches to mapping inequalities in mental health has been the split in the literature between studies of the social determinants of mental health problems and studies of inequalities in access to care. Hollingshead and Redlich's classic text *Social Class and Mental Illness* explored levels of identified mental disorder in the community, pathways to service provision and treatment of mental health problems. The rhetoric of contemporary epidemiology certainly emphasises the importance of collecting information in a defined geographical area, in order to estimate the extent of unmet need and calculate the services required in order to meet it.

However, whilst on the face of things there has been some recognition of the connectedness between the identification of patterns of mental health problems at a population level and service provision, analytically this has been limited. Little social psychiatric epidemiology extends beyond a view about the services required to meet 'need', such as the provision of a specified number of beds or outpatient or day hospital places. In other words, the nature and purpose of services is framed only within the terms of psychiatric treatment and case management and does not address aspects of social need or social exclusion.

An important implication of the last point is that a medicalised view of mental illness encourages an assumption that the provision of services should simply parallel that for physical illness. In Chapter 3, when discussing the inverse care law, we noted that the translation of a 'greater access for those in most need' philosophy from physical to mental health care has been problematic. The association of mental health service provision with coercion and the failure to meet expressed need puts an altogether different gloss on obtaining 'equality of access' for those with mental health problems.

Causes of mental health problems and their management have generally been considered as separate domains in the study of mental health inequalities. The categorical and normative reasoning, which has characterised psychiatric knowledge, has been compounded by a failure to question the role that service provision has had in either generating or ameliorating inequalities.

One aspect of contemporary service provision is its failure to address the social influences and wider social context of those who present with mental health need and are 'treated' by services. We have shown at various points in this book how being diagnosed with a mental health problem leads to social rejection and the internalisation of stigma, which results in a poor quality of life and permanent exclusion from mainstream social institutions and everyday life. Much of the problem lies in a failure to incorporate a robust view of social inclusion between service and non-service boundaries into mainstream mental health provision. Research findings demonstrating that suicide amongst young men and violent incidents involving those with mental health problems are most likely to occur in the days and weeks following psychiatric discharge highlight this disconnection between service provision and the outside world.

In the past, service provision based on a social model of mental health placed social divisions centre-stage. Epistemological countercurrents to the medical model were evident from the 1960s onwards. Radicalised object-relations theory was utilised to link individual distress to its outer social roots. These and other theories were made manifest in key practical projects which lay outside the hierarchical, doctor-centred State service. These included many projects which still make an important contribution but are not often given a high profile (such as the Philadelphia and Arbours Associations and Women's Therapy Centres). In the voluntary sector, MIND and the Richmond Fellowship still contribute to the material and social needs of clients through a network of residential and non-residential services.

These projects, added to in recent years by service models based on alternative knowledge and practices associated with the rise of the users' movement, demonstrate that in a British context a less medical and more social approach to service delivery is possible. However, whilst such social models exist, they have not been fully incorporated into mainstream services. This is not through a failure to recognise the importance of social influences. Contemporary UK mental health policy addresses these issues explicitly and has highlighted the need for public health approaches to mental health policy and the need for other sectors such as primary care to become more involved as a means of addressing the root causes of social disadvantage and mental health (see Chapter 4). However, policy in the UK, which incorporates action to address social inclusion, is currently aspirational. Key impediments to implementation are evident which tend not to be acknowledged in official policy statements. We have shown how in relation to primary care, despite an acknowledgement of the social influences and models in relation to mental health, there remain problems about progressing beyond an individualised level.

Our focus on primary care in Chapter 4 sought to explore the recursive relationship between service contact and the construction of a particular gendered and individualised view of life problems and psychological distress emanating from peoples' personal and social situations. We attempted to illuminate the way in which the recognition of the social origins of mental illness and a public health response to dealing with mental health problems within primary care has been subtly and inadvertently thwarted by common practices adopted by professionals. The latter are, to a large extent, shaped by organisational constraints and external influences, such as drug-company activity.

An increasingly common consensual view between patients and practitioners exists that 'depression' emanates from personal and social conditions and is inadequately dealt with by a technical, medicalised response. However, both parties find it easier to perpetuate rather than challenge this response. In part, this is because of a sense of a lack of professional control over the socio-economic causes of mental distress and the relative absence of effective clinical (i.e., individually targeted) interventions. Additionally, within a medical culture of primary care, mental health does not have the same salience, or attractiveness, as more coherent clinical entities such as coronary heart disease (also the target of centrally driven policies to reverse inequalities). Thus, in relative terms, there is an inertia which contributes to the marginalisation of mental health in the culture of primary care work. The result is one in which, currently, there is little room for manoeuvre for primary care professionals beyond reinforcing a medicalised and individualised response to social injury.

The demands for a new 'primary-care-led' health policy do not acknowledge the countervailing forces, which act to promote an individualised medicalised response at the expense of approaches that seek to address social exclusion and disadvantage. For example, little official comment has been noted about the activities of drug companies or the negative and iatrogenic effects of drug companies which manufacture psychotropic drugs. The interests of the State are heavily bound up with developing a positive relationship with drug companies, for economic reasons, which extend beyond the boundaries of the health services. Thus, one of the major questions which arises is the extent to which official government policies in advanced welfare capitalist societies are able, effectively and meaningfully, to promote a policy agenda about tackling social exclusion without identifying and opposing those vested interests which undermine its intentions.

In Chapter 5, we explored life-course effects and showed that inequality needs to be understood in a longitudinal as well as cross-sectional way. There are 'constants' across time which vary in their salience – good physical health, high socio-economic status, benign/supportive personal relationships and positive coping strategies all predict and constitute good mental health at any age. However, childhood is a particularly vulnerable period in two senses: average levels of mental distress are at their highest in young people; and early social insults (poverty, neglect and abuse) predict poor mental health in later life. The balance between social conformity and personal autonomy creates stressors which are peculiar to middle adulthood. In old age, physical health becomes a particularly important mediator of mental health. A potential feedback or reinforcing link with patterns of help-seeking and service contact is also a consideration at different points in the life-span. For teenagers, a lack of confidence and insecure identity may coalesce with perceptions of services as stigmatising, which may lead to a failure to provide support at a time where school attainment is likely to influence life chances.

By the time we reached Chapter 6, we could place a central theme about the psychiatric patient in society (a reputation for dangerousness) into a wider context. The workings of the mental health industry are shaped in part by a number of contextualising factors: public prejudice; vote-sensitive governments; and the individualisation of social processes. The investigation of violence can expose these workings by encouraging us to examine people with mental health problems as victims, rather than as perpetrators, of violence. Indeed, there is much stronger evidence to support the idea that violence generates mental distress than the assumption that people with mental health problems are unusually dangerous. By reframing the question of the relationship between violence and mental health problems, we glimpse the political interests at work in the dynamics of warfare. We also glimpse the advantages to those in power of the social exclusion and demonisation of people with mental health problems.

Chapter 7 drew attention to the relationship between the knowledge-base of the mental health professions, particularly psychiatry, and power. We explored how knowledge is bound up with gaining and retaining power over colleagues in competing professions and patients. Also, knowledge claims may illuminate or obscure the social context of power relationships. In the field of mental health, knowledge-in-action is intimately linked to social regulation and so it provides a normative function. With this normative role of the 'psy complex' comes an inevitable individualisation of distress and a tendency towards either biological or psychological reductionism.

Lay knowledge, with its focus on experiential knowledge, identity and the connection between social conditions and personal troubles, has acted as a counter to this and provides an alternative basis upon which to provide a response to social exclusion and disadvantage. However, such an approach is likely to come up against a more established and entrenched professional knowledge-base and practice.

In Chapter 8, we discussed the impact of the negative experiences of the 'older' psychotropic medications reported by users. A new generation of drugs may have the potential to bring about fewer 'side-effects', which in turn has implications for social functioning and reduction in stigma.

Given the biological bias of the psychiatric profession explored episodically in the book, Chapter 8 condensed a set of criticisms about biological interventions from both mental health professionals and service users. We noted that the dominance of drug treatments has created a sort of imposed pseudo-democracy, with most patients receiving drugs whether they want them are not. This pseudo-democracy has led to users resenting their lack of choice and their relatives complaining that some drugs are not offered because of their cost. For many psychiatrists, treatment has simply come to mean medication. A similar assumption is made by politicians, when they seek legal powers to ensure treatment compliance. Neither of these parties places concerns about iatrogenic damage high on their agenda, nor are they overly concerned about what patients might tell them about such damage.

Given the resentment expressed by service users about physical treatments, there has been a tendency for them to turn to talking treatments for a more humane response from professionals. However, in Chapter 9 we introduced a number of cautions about this preference. Talking treatments are not offered equally to people. Moreover, as with physical treatment, they can create iatrogenic damage. Thus, although the availability of talking treatments is differentially offered (to the rich, white people, women and younger adults), it is not clear whether those excluded should be resentful.

Our approach to mental health and inequality has sought to make conceptual links across a range of domains (e.g., service provision, knowledge and wider social influences). The intention has been to begin to provide a broader theoretical basis from which to understand the nature and complexity of social disadvantage and exclusion and its association with mental health. The evidence and links we have made in the different chapters of this book point to the need to develop further models of analysis and forms of therapeutic practice which link individual distress to its social context. Specifically, mental health policy needs to set, as an explicit aim, changes in the social environment as a whole which would reverse the exclusion of those people experiencing or being vulnerable to mental health problems from economic and social life. Our analysis points unambiguously to the need for mental health services to facilitate social inclusion.

Notes

Introduction

1 In official British policy-making circles during the 1980s and early 1990s, there was a preference for the term 'variation' rather than 'inequality'.

2 Thus, some of us start from the belief that we are all 'equal before God'. Others, such as meritocratic social democrats and liberals, may believe in the importance of 'equality of opportunity', whilst socialists may emphasise an incremental or revolutionary reduction in income and power differentials. All of these may believe (rightly or wrongly) that equality of access to health care will reduce inequalities in health. Some, following Durkheim and Parsons, emphasise that for society to function there *have to be* inequalities of status, class and income in order to maintain norms through rewards for those conforming to, and punishments or disincentives for those deviating from, social expectations. This normative view has a particular relevance for people with mental health problems, because they are considered to have violated an implicit social contract by rule breaking and role failure.

3 John Pilger, in a piece on Australian poverty in his set of political essays, *A Secret Country*, cites Jules Feiffer when making this point: 'I used to think I was poor. Then they told me I wasn't poor I was needy. Then they told me it was self-defeating to think of myself of needy. I was deprived. Then they told me deprived was a bad image. I was underprivileged. Then they told me underprivileged was over used. I was disadvantaged. I still don't have a cent. But I have a great vocabulary' (Feiffer cited in Pilger 1989: 313).

4 Carried out at the National Primary Care Research and Development Centre at the University of Manchester.

Chapter 1   Epidemiology and its limits

1 There are a number of very useful texts which summarise and analyse the extensive evidence on mental health inequalities. These include a book summarising research on social injury, *Adversity, Stress and Psychopathology*, Dohrenwend, B.P. (1998) (Oxford: Oxford University Press). This

provides excellent sections on extreme situation, individual events, epidemiological and case control studies, stress moderating and amplifying factors and complementary approaches.

2 Examples of overviews of key evidence about social class include the following articles: Muntaner, C., Eaton, W.W., Diala, C., Kessler, R.C. and Sorlie, P.D. (1998) 'Social class, assets, organisational control and prevalence of common groups of psychiatric disorders', *Social Science and Medicine*, vol. 47, pp. 2043–53; Weich, S. and Lewis, G. (1998) 'Material standard of living, social class and the prevalence of the common mental disorders in Great Britain', *Journal of Epidemiology and Community Health*, vol. 52, pp. 8–14; Lewis, G., Bebbington, P., Brugha, T., Farrell, M., Gill, B., Jenkins, R. and Meltzer, H. (1998) 'Socio-economic status, standard of living and neurotic disorder', *Lancet*, vol. 352, pp. 605–9.

3 Whilst we refer at different points in this book to a range of evidence which relates to gender and mental health, for a summary and overview the following are useful texts: see, for example, Dohrenwend, B.P. and Dohrenwend, B.S. (1976) 'Sex differences and psychiatric disorders', *American Journal of Sociology*, vol. 6, pp. 1447–54; Ussher, J. (1991) *Womens's Madness: Misogyny or Mental Illness?* (London: Harvester-Wheatsheaf); Russell, D. (1995) *Women, Madness and Medicine* (Oxford: Polity); Rosenfeld, S. (1999) 'Gender and Mental Health: Do women have more psychopathology, men more or both the same?', in Horowitz, A. and Scheid, T. (eds), (1998) *A Handbook for the Study of Mental Health* (Cambridge: Cambridge University Press).

4 See, for example, Fernando, S. (1988) *Race and Culture in Psychiatry* (London: Tavistock Routledge) for an overview and Williams, D. and Harris-Reid, M. (1999) 'Race and Mental Health: emerging patterns and promising approaches', in Horowitz and Scheid (eds), *Handbook for the Study of Mental Health*; Dohrenwend *et al.* (1998) 'Ethnicity: socioeconomic status and psychiatric disorders: a test of the social causation–social selection issue', in Dohrenwend, B.P. (ed.), *Adversity, Stress and Psychopathology*.

5 Vulnerability factors refer to both personal and environmental influences (e.g., loss of mother before 11 years, lack of employment outside the home). Provoking agents are factors operating in women's contemporary everyday lives, including detrimental events such as loss through bereavement or marriage breakdown, or episodes of serious illness. Chronic difficulties as well as specific stressors are also included. Symptom formation factors refer to previous episodes of depression and personal characteristics such as low self-esteem.

6 Hollingshead and Redlich's epidemiological survey published in 1958 included an appendix containing data on sex differences.

7 Note it is '*the* pathophysiology of schizophrenia' (the definite article implying a definitive statement and an established certainty). And the notion of 'a physical basis' alluded to by Csernansky and Grace is so broad that it cannot be wrong – there is a 'physical basis' for *all* behaviour and experience, normal or abnormal, because the brain is always implicated in human functioning. In the rhetoric of biological psychiatry,

'physical' or 'biological' elide, over and over again, into 'pathological'. When physiology for medicine becomes 'pathophysiology', an amalgam statement of epistemological jurisdiction and professional power is being made.

8   Hospital rundown occurred in many countries before neuroleptics were introduced and they were given enthusiastically to groups other than those with a diagnosis of schizophrenia (agitated older people and those with learning disabilities).

9   The prescribing of antidepressants for vague symptoms in the absence of a formal diagnostic label of depression is a further indication of a normalising tendency in relation to depression, as is the widespread acceptance in the media and popular press of a normalised view of depression.

Chapter 2   Neighbourhood, community and mental health

1   Compositional effects are those influences that might be derived from the collective effect of individuals who are disadvantaged at an individual level (e.g., those on low incomes) living in disadvantaged areas. Contextual effects refer to specific features and the nature of the neighbourhood.

2   This concept has its roots in Durkheim's analysis of the presence or absence of societal norms as a principal explanatory factor in suicidal conduct. The stronger the forces which throw individuals back on their own resources, the greater the rate of suicide. Where there is close integration of the individual with collective life, the rate of suicide is lower.

3   Peter Huxley, Sherril Evans, Claire Gately, Richard Thomas and Brian Robson.

4   Modified labelling theory according to (Link *et al.* 1989) suggests a causal role for stigma in relapse as a result of spoiled identity linked to negative outcomes in employment and social functioning etc. The effects of 'labelling' are mediated by social psychological mechanisms in which both ex-mental patients and members of the general population internalise negative cultural conceptions and negative attitudes about 'the mentally ill' which lead to personal discrimination.

5   Its inclusion alongside coronary heart disease, cancer and older people is a sign of mental health's integration within a broad health and welfare agenda for recent 'New Labour' governments.

Chapter 3   Inequalities created by service provision

1   Drawn from the *Diagnostic and Statistical Manual of the American Psychiatric Association*, 3rd edition, as revised.

Chapter 4 Primary care, mental health and inequalities

1 Where estimates suggest that 80 per cent of those who might be considered by clinical standards to be suffering from PND do not report with symptoms to any health professional.
2 Type 1 evidence: systematic reviews including RCTs; Type II evidence: minimum of one 'good' RCT; Type III evidence: minimum of one 'well designed' interventions study without randomisation; Type IV evidence: at least one well designed observational study; Type V evidence: expert opinion 'including the opinion of services users and carers'.
3 This is illustrated by the comments of the authors of a recent systematic review of psychosocial mental health who concluded that 'current research into psychosocial treatments reflects different levels of quality of evidence and an increasing but *only* partially achieved picture of well targeted and well evaluated interventions' p. 173 McGorry *et al.* 1997).
4 Williams, B., Coyle, J., Healy, D. (1998) The meaning of patient satisfaction: an explanation of high reported levels. *Social Science and Medicine.* vol. 47, pp. 1351–9.

Chapter 5 Influences on mental health inequalities across the life-span

1 Not only is there a relationship between low educational attainment and behavioural difficulties which is socially patterned (according to ethnicity and gender), but evidence of the direct effects of school functioning and ethos on mental health outcomes (Mortimor *et al.* 1988; Rutter *et al.* 1979).
2 Raviv *et al.* (2000) found that adolescents were far more willing to refer to another person other than themselves in their accounts of personal problem and help-seeking was considered in terms of a 'threat to self-mechanism'. A reluctance of ethnic minority groups to seek help has also been noted (Saunders *et al.* 1994).

Chapter 6 Violence: victimhood and discrimination

1 The four methodological problems are:
• *Inadequacy of predictors* – Although the genesis of violence implicates many social, psychological and biological factors, research has been overly restrictive in its attention to just a few predictive variables such as psychiatric diagnosis, history of violence and substance abuse (Monahan and Steadman 1994).
• *Weak criterion variables* – Different studies use different criteria to define violent outcomes and vary in their validation of these measures.

- *Constricted validation samples* – Some social groups (such as psychiatric patients and prisoners) have been subject to intense scrutiny but there has been a poor recruitment of larger population samples (McNiel *et al*. 1988; Teplin 1990). Also, the environmental frame of the research needs to be taken into consideration. Monahan (2000) notes that studying inpatients in highly structured environments with intense staff scrutiny probably artificially *lowers* the base rate of violence. A bias in the other direction occurs in community samples, where non-patient groups, with their own base rate of violence, are studied less than patient groups.
- *Unsynchronised research efforts* – Research on violence and mental disorder has entailed predictor and criterion variables being defined idiosyncratically. As a result, a comparison of the results and interpretation from different studies is difficult. Thus, much research has been done on the topic but overall conclusions are not always readily drawn.
2 Take the example of paedophilia. The logic surrounding the diagnosis of psychology, goes like this: Q. Why do some men molest children? A. Because they are psychopaths. Q. How do we know they are psychopaths? A. Because they molest children.

Chapter 7   Professional and lay knowledge

1 User satisfaction surveys have further limitations insofar as they may not recognise the nature of service provision over time and the subjective impact that this may have. Negative experiences of service contact are internalised subjectively. This is clearly seen in relation to recent research on Afro-Caribbean people who, as we have seen above, are subject to more coercive treatment. Black patients (who had received a label of psychotic disorder), most notably those of second generation born in the UK, were significantly less satisfied with almost every aspect of the services they received than either older Afro-Caribbean patients born in the Caribbean or white patients. The number of previous admissions was found to be a significant predictor of satisfaction (Parkman *et al.* 1997).

Chapter 8   Biological treatments: a case of imposed equality

1 The growth in over-the-counter products allows those with the financial resources autonomously to manage their own conditions more than those who lack such financial means.
2 Psychiatrists who have self-administered phenothiazines, even in low doses, have reported dramatically distressing experiences in relation to akathisia and dysphoria.

3 Organisations such as the National Institute for Clinical Excellence are charged with making recommendations about what should be provided by the NHS in part as a response to the inequities that arose from rationing decisions made by individual health authorities.

References

Abood, L. (1960) 'A chemical approach to the problem of mental disease', in D. Jackson (ed.), *The Etiology of Schizophrenia* (New York: Basic Books).

Acierno, R., Byre, C., Resnick, H.S. and Kilpatrick, D.G. (1998) 'Adult victims of physical violence', in A.S. Bellack and M. Hersen (eds), *Comprehensive Clinical Psychology vol. 9 Applications in Diverse Populations* (London: Pergamon).

Agnew, R. (1999) 'A general strain theory of community differences in crime rates', *Journal of Research in Crime and Delinquency*, vol. 36, pp. 123–55.

Aldarondo, E. (1998) 'Perpetrators of Domestic Violence', in A.S. Bellack and M. Hersen (eds), *Comprehensive Clinical Psychology vol. 9 Applications in Diverse Populations* (London: Pergamon).

Alzeimer's Disease Report (1992) (London: Alzheimer's Disease Society).

American Psychiatric Association DSM III (1980) *Diagnostic and Statistical Manual for Mental Disorders* (New York: American Psychiatric Association).

Anderson, J., Martin, J., Mullen, P., Romans, S. and Herbison, P. (1993) 'Prevalence of childhood sexual abuse in a community sample of women', *Journal of American Academy of Child and Adolescent Psychiatry*, vol. 32, pp. 911–19.

Andrulis, D. (1998) 'Access to care is the centrepiece in the elimination of socio-economic disparities in health', *Annals of Internal Medicine*, vol. 129, no. 5, pp. 412–16.

Aneshensel, C.S. (1992) 'Social stress theory and research', *Annual Review of Sociology*, vol. 18, pp. 15–58.

Anehensel, C.S. and Succoff, S. (1996) 'The neighbourhood context of adolescent mental health', *Journal of Health and Social Behaviour*, vol. 37, pp. 293–311.

Annadale, E. and Hunt, K. (eds), (2000), *Gender Inequalities in Health* (Buckingham: Open University Press).

Applebaum, P.S., Robbins, P.C. and Roth, L.H. (1999) 'A dimensional approach to delusions: comparisons across delusion type and diagnoses', *American Journal of Psychiatry*, vol. 156, pp. 1938–43.

Appleby, L., Shaw, J., Amos, T., McDonnell, R.M., Harris, C., McCann, K., Davies, S., Buckly, H. and Parsons, R. (1999) '"Suicide with 12 months off" contact with mental health services: National clinical survey', *British Medical Journal*, vol. 318, pp. 1235–9.

Baldessarini, R.J. (1999) 'Psychopharmacology', in A.M. Nicholi (ed.), *The Harvard Guide to Psychiatry* (London: Harvard University Press).

Bannister, D. (1983) 'The internal politics of psychotherapy', in D. Pilgrim (ed.), *Psychology and Psychotherapy* (London: Routledge).

Barham, P. and Haywood, R. (1991) *From the Mental Patient to the Person* (London: Routledge).

Barnes, A. and Ephross, P.H. (1994) 'The impact of hate violence on victims. Emotional and behavioral responses to attacks', *Social Work*, vol. 39, pp. 247–51.

Barnes, M. (1999) 'Users as citizens: Collective action and the local governance of welfare', *Social Policy and Administration*, vol. 33, no. 1, pp. 73–90 (Mar.).

Barnes, M. and Maple, N. (1992) *Women and Mental Health: Challenging the Stereotypes* (Birmingham: Venture Press).

Barrett, A.E. (2000) 'Marital trajectories and mental health', *Journal of Health and Social Behavior*, vol. 41, pp. 451–64.

Bartels, J. *et al.* (1991) 'Characteristic hostility, in schizophrenic outpatients', *schizophrenia Bulletin*, vol. 17, pp. 163–71.

Bartley, M., Blane, D. and Davey Smith, G. (1998) 'Introduction: beyond the Black Report', *Sociology of Health and Illness*, vol. 20, no. 5, pp. 563–78.

Barton, W.R. (1958) *Institutional Neurosis* (Bristol: Wright & Sons).

Baruch, G. and Treacher, A. (1978) *Psychiatry Observed* (London: Routledge).

Basaglia, F. (1981) 'Breaking the circuit of control', in D. Ingleby (ed.) *Critical Psychiatry* (Harmondsworth: Penguin).

Bassuk, E.L. and Geerson, S. (1978) 'Deinstitutionalisation and mental health services', *Scientific American*, vol. 238, no. 2, pp. 46–53.

Baxter, D. and Appleby, L. (1999) 'Case register study of suicide risk in mental disorders', *British Journal of Psychiatry*, vol. 175, pp. 32–326.

Bean, P. (1980) *Compulsory Admissions to Mental Hospital* (London: Wiley).

Bean, P. (1986) *Mental Disorder and Legal Control* (Cambridge: Cambridge University Press).

Bean, P. and Mounser, P. (1993) *Discharged from Mental Hospitals* (London: Macmillan).

Bebbington, P., Christopher, T. and Hurry, J. (1981) 'Adversity and the nature of psychiatric disorders in the community', *Journal of Affective Disorders*, vol. 3, pp. 345–66.

Becker, D. (2000) 'When she was bad: borderline personality disorder in a posttraumatic age', *Amercial Journal of Orthopsychiatry*, vol. 70, no. 4, pp. 422–31.

Bentall, R.P., Jackson, H. and Pilgrim, D. (1988) 'Abandoning the concept of schizophrenia; some implications of validity arguments for psychological research into psychosis', *British Journal of Clinical Psychology*, vol. 27, pp. 305–24.

Benton, T. (1991) 'Biology and social science: why a return of the repressed should be given a (cautious) welcome', *Sociology*, vol. 25, pp. 1–29.

Berrigan, L.P. and Garfield, S. (1981) 'Relationship of missed psychotherapy appointments to premature termination and social class', *British Journal of Clinical Psychology*, vol. 20, pp. 239–42.

Bhaskar, R. (1989) *Reclaiming Reality: A Critical Introduction to Contemporary Philosophy* (London: Verso).

Bhaskar, R. (1998) *The Possibility of Naturalism: A Philosophical Critique of the Contemporary Human Science* (London: Routledge).

Bhugra, D. and Jones, P. (2001) 'Migration and mental health', *Advances in Psychiatric Treatment*, vol. 7, no. 3, pp. 216–23.

Bifulco, A., Bernazzini, O., Moran, P.M. and Ball, C. (2000) 'Lifetime stressors and recurrent depression: preliminary findings of the adult life phase interview', *Social Psychiatry and Psychiatric Epidemiology*, vol. 35, pp. 264–75.

Bion, W. (1977) *Seven Servants* (New York: Jason Aranson).

Bird, H., Canino, G., Rubio-Stipec, M., Gould, M.S., Ribera, J.C., Sesman, M., Woodbery, M., Heutos-Goldman, S., Pagan, A., Sanchez-Lakey, A. and Moscosco, M. (1988) 'Estimates of the prevalence of childhood maladjustment in a community survey in Puerto Rico', *Archives of General Psychiatry*, vol. 43, pp. 1120–26.

Blackburn, I.M., Bishop, S., Glen, A.I., Whalley, L.J. and Christie, J.E. (1981) 'The efficacy of cognitive therapy in depression', *British Journal of Psychiatry*, vol. 139, pp. 181–9.

Blacker, D. and Tsuang, M.T. (1999) 'Classification and DSM-IV', in A.M. Nicholi (ed.) *The Harvard Guide to Psychiatry* (3rd edn) (London: Belknap).

Blane, D. (1995) 'Social determinants of health, socio-economic status, social class ethnicity', *American Journal of Public Health*, vol. 85, pp. 903–4.

Blane, D.B., Bartley, M. and Davey Smith, G. (1997) 'Disease etiology and materialist explanations of socio-economic mortality differentials', *European Journal of Public Health*, vol. 7, pp. 385–91.

Blaxter, M. (1990) *Health and Lifestyles* (London: Routledge).

Blazer, D.G. (1994) 'Epidemiology of late-life depression', in I.S. Schneider *et al.* (eds) *Diagnosis and Treatment of Depression in Late Life* (Washington DC: American Psychiatry Press).

Bloch, S. and Reddaway, P. (1977) *Psychiatric Terror* (London: Routledge).

Blumenthal, S. and Lavender, T. (2000) *Violence and Mental Disorder: A Critical Aid to the Assessment and Management of Risk* (London: Zito Trust).

Bowlby, J. (1951) *Maternal Care and Mental Health* (Geneva: World Health Organization).

Boyle, M. (1990) *Schizophrenia: A Scientific Delusion?* (London: Routledge).

Boyle, R.J., Gattrell, A.C. and Duke-Williams, G. (1999) 'The effect on morbidity of variability in deprivation and population stability in England and Wales: an investigation at small area level', *Social Science and Medicine*, vol. 49, pp. 791–9.

Boyne, R. (1990) *Foucault and Derrida: The Other Side of Reason* (London: Unwin Hyman).

Braam, A.W., Beckman, A.T.F., van Tilburg, Deeg, D.G.H. and van Tilburg, W. (1997) 'Religious involvement and depression in older Dutch citizens', *Social Psychiatry and Psychiatric Epidemiology*, vol. 32, pp. 284–91.

Braceland, I. (1977) 'Psychiatry and the third revolution', *Psychiatric Annals*, vol. 7, no. 10, pp. 4–5.

Bracken, P. and Thomas, P. (1998) 'A new debate in mental health', *Open Mind*, vol. 89, p. 17.

Brayne, C. and Ames, D. (1988) 'The epidemiology of mental disorders in old age', in B. Gearing, M. Johnson and T. Heller (eds) *Mental Health Problems in Old Age* (London: Wiley).

Breggin, P. (1993) *Toxic Psychiatry* (London: Fontana).

Briere, J. and Runtz, M. (1987) 'Post-sexual abuse trauma: data implications for clinical practice', *Journal of Interpersonal Violence*, vol. 2, pp. 367–79.

Brown, G.W. and Harris, T. (1978) *The Social Origins of Depression* (London: Tavistock).

Brown, G.W., Harris, T. and Hepworth, C. (1995) 'Loss, humiliation and entrapment among women developing depression: a patient and non-patient comparison', *Psychological Medicine*, vol. 25, pp. 7–21.

Brown, G.W. and Moran, P.M. (1997) 'Single mothers, poverty and depression', *Psychological Medicine*, vol. 27, pp. 21–33.

Brown, G.W. and Wing, J.K. (1962) 'A comparative clinical social survey of three mental hospitals', *The Sociological Review Monograph*, vol. 5, pp. 145–71.

Brown, P. (1992) 'Popular Epidemiology and Toxic-Waste Contamination – lay and professional ways of knowing', *Journal of Health and Social Behaviour*, vol. 33, no. 3, pp. 267–81.

Brown, P. and Funk, S.C. (1986) 'Tardive dyskinesia: barriers to the professional recognition of iatrogenic disease', *Journal of Health and Social Behaviour*, vol. 27, pp. 116–32.

Browne, A. and Williams, K.R. (1993) 'Gender, intimacy and lethal violence; trends from 1976–1987', *Gender and Society*, vol. 7, pp. 78–98.

Bruce, M.L. (1998) 'Divorce and psychopathology', in B.P. Dohrenwend (ed.) *Adversity, Stress and Psychopathology* (Oxford: Oxford University Press).

Buchanan, A. (1999) *What Works for Troubles Children?* (London: Barnados).

Buck, N., Gershuny, J., Rose, D. and Scott, J. (1994) *Changing Households: The British Household Panel Survey 1990–1992* (Colchester: ESRC Research Centre on Micro-Social Change).

Burchell, B. (1992) 'Towards a social psychology of the labour market', *Journal of Occupational and Organisational Psychology*, vol. 65, pp. 345–54.

Busfield, J. (1994) 'Is mental illness a female malady? Men, women and madness in nineteenth century England', *Sociology*, vol. 28, pp. 259–77.

Cahill, J. (1983) 'Structure characteristics of the macro-economy and mental health', *American Journal of Community Psychology*, vol. 11, pp. 553–71.

Campbell, M., Rapoport, J. and Simpson, G.M. (1999) 'Antipsychotics in children and adolescents', *Journal of the American Academy of Child and Adolescent Psychiatry*, vol. 38, no. 5, pp. 537–45.

Carpenter, J. and Sbaraini, S. (1997) *Choice Information and Dignity: Involving Users and Carers in Care Management in Mental Health* (London: Policy Press).

Carpenter, M. (2000) ' "It's a small world" mental health policy under welfare capitalism since 1945', *Sociology of Health and Illness*, vol. 22, no. 5, pp. 602–19.

Chamberlin, J. (1988) *On Our Own* (London: Mind Publications).

Chasseguet-Smirgel, J. and Grunberger, B. (1986) *Freud or Reich: Psychoanalysis and Illusion* (London: Free Associations Books).

Cheng, A.T.A. (2001) 'Case definition and culture: are people all the same?', *British Journal of Psychiatry*, vol. 179, pp. 1–3.

Chesler, P. (1972) *Women and Madness* (New York: Doubleday).

Chodorow, N. (1978) *The Reproduction of Mothering* (London: University of California Press).

Clare, A. (1977) *Psychiatry in Dissent* (London: Tavistock).

Clare, A. (1979) Review of *Psychiatry Observed* by Baruch and Treacher, in *Psychological Medicine*, vol. 9, pp. 387–9.

Clare, A. (1999) 'Psychiatry's future: psychological medicine or biological psychiatry?', *Journal of Mental Health*, vol. 8, no. 2, pp. 109–11.

Clark, C. and Mezey, G. (1997) 'Elderly offenders against children', *Journal of Forensic Psychiatry*, vol. 8, no. 2, pp. 357–69.

Clark, D.E. and Wildner, M. (2000) 'Violence and fear of violence in East and West Germany', *Social Science and Medicine*, vol. 51, pp. 373–79.

Clayton, P.J. (1986) 'Bereavement and its relationship to clinical depression', in H. Hippius (ed.) *New Results in Depression* (Berlin: Springer Verlag).

Clayton, P.J. (1998) 'The model of stress: the bereavement reaction', in B.P. Dohrenwend (ed.) *Adversity, Stress and Psychopathology* (Oxford: Oxford University Press).

Cochrane, R. and Bal, S. (1989) 'Mental hospital admission rates of immigrants to England: a comparison of 1971 and 1981', *Social Psychiatry*, vol. 24, pp. 2–11.

Cohen, D. (1997) 'A critique of the use of neuroleptic drugs in psychiatry', in S. Fisher and R.P. Greenberg (eds) *From Placebo to Panacea* (New York: Wiley).

Cole, M.G. and Bellevance, F. (1997) 'Depression in elderly inpatients: a meta-analysis of outcomes', *Canadian Medical Association Journal*, vol. 157, pp. 1055–60.

Commander, M.J., Dharan, S.P., Odell, S.M. and Surtees, P.C. (1997a) 'Access to mental health care in an inner-city health district, I: pathways into and within specialist psychiatric services', *British Journal of Psychiatry*, vol. 170, pp. 312–16.

Commander, M.J., Dharan, S.P., Odell, S.M. and Surtees, P.C. (1997b) 'Access to mental health care in an inner-city health district, II: Association with demographic factors', *British Journal of Psychiatry*, vol. 170, pp. 317–20.

Conrad, P. and Schneider, J.W. (1985) *Deviance and Medicalisation* (Columbus, OH: Merril).

Cooper, B. (1989) 'The epidemiological contribution to research on late-life dementia', in P. Williams, G. Wilkinson and K. Rawnsley (eds) *The Scope of Epidemiological Psychiatry* (London: Routledge).

Copeland, J., Dewey, M., Wodd, N. *et al.* (1987) 'Range of mental illness among the elderly in the community', *British Journal of Psychiatry*, vol. 150, pp. 815–23.

Costello, E.J., Edelbrook, C.S., Costello, A.J., Dulcan, M.K., Burns, B. and Brent, D. (1988) 'Psychiatric disorder in paediatric primary care: the new hidden morbidity', *Paediatrics*, vol. 82, pp. 415–24.

Coulter, J. (1973) *Approaches to Insanity* (London: Martin Robinson).

Craig, K.M. and Waldo, C.R. (1996) ' "So what's a hate crime anyway?": young adults perceptions of hate crimes, victims and perpetrators', *Law and Human Behavior*, vol. 20, pp. 113–29.

Crepaz-Keay, D., Binns, C. and Wilson, E. (1998) *Dancing with Angels: Involving Survivors in Mental Health Training* (London: CCETSW).

Crossley, M.L., and Crossley, N. (2001) '"Patient" voices, social movements and the habitus: how psychiatric survivors "speak out" ', *Social Science and Medicine*, vol. 52, no. 10, pp. 1477–89.

Crossley, N. (1998) 'Transforming the mental health field: the early history of the National Association for Mental Health', *Sociology of Health and Illness*, vol. 20, no. 4, pp. 458–88.

Csernansky, J.G. and Grace, A.A. (1998) 'New models of the pathophysiology of schizophrenia', *Schizophrenia Bulletin*, vol. 24, no. 2, pp. 185–8.

Currer, C. (1986) 'Concepts of well- and ill-being: the case of Pathan mothers on Britain', in C. Currer and M. Stacey (eds) *Concepts of Health Illness and Disease* (Leamington Spa: Berg).

Curtis, S. and Rees-Jones, I. (1998) 'In there a place for geography in the analysis of health inequality?', *Sociology of Health and Illness*, vol. 20, no. 5, pp. 546–673.

Dadds, M.R., Sanders, M.R., Morrison, M. and Rebgetz, M. (1992). 'Childhood depression and conduct disorder, II: an analysis of family interaction patterns in the home', *Journal of Abnormal Psychology*, vol. 101, pp. 505–13.

Dallaire, B., McGubbin, M., Morin, P. and Cohen, D. (2000) 'Civil commitment due to mental illness and dangerousness: the union of law and psychiatry within a treatment-control system', *Sociology of Health and Illness*, vol. 22, no. 5, pp. 679–99.

Daniels, H., Visser, J., Cole, T. and deReybekill, N. (1999) *Emotional and Behavioural Difficulties in Mainstream Schools* (London: Department of Education and Employment).

Davidson, J. (2000) 'A phenomenology of fear: Merleau-Ponty and agoraphobic life-worlds', *Sociology of Health and Illness*, vol. 22, no. 5, pp. 640–60.

Dean, P.J. and Range, L.M. (1999) 'Testing the escape theory of suicide in an outpatient clinical population', *Cognitive Therapy and Research*, vol. 23, pp. 561–72.

Dear, M. and Laws, G. (1986) 'Anatomy of a decision: recent land zoning appeals and their effect on group home locations in Ontario', *Canadian Journal of Community Health*, vol. 5, pp. 5–17.

Dear, M. and Wolch, J. (1987) *Landscapes of Despair: From Institutionalisation to Homelessness* (Oxford: Polity Press).

de Swann, A. (1990) *The Management of Normality* (London: Routledge).

DHSS (1980) *Inequalities in Health: Report of a Working Group* (London: HMSO).

Dixon, C. (2000) 'A multi-method evaluation of a training package for GPs in the assessment and management of depression' (Unpublished Ph.D thesis, University of Manchester).

DoH (1998a) *Modernising Mental Health Services: Safe, Sound and Supportive* (London: Stationery Office).

DoH (1998b) *Our Healthier Nation* (London: Stationery Office).
DoH (1999) *A National Service Framework for Mental Health* (London: Stationery Office).
DoH (2000) *A National Service Framework for Coronary Heart Disease* (London: Stationery Office).
DoH (2001) *The Mental Health Policy Implementation Guide* (London: Stationery Office).
Dohrenwend, B.P. (1990a) 'Socio-economic status (SES) and psychiatric disorders: are the issues still compelling?', *Social Psychiatry and Psychiatric Epidemiology*, vol. 25, pp. 41–7.
Dohrenwend, B.P. (1990b) 'The problem of validity in field studies of psychological disorders revisited', *Psychological Medicine*, vol. 20, pp. 195–208.
Dohrenwend, B.P. (1998) 'A psychosocial perspective on the past and future of psychiatric epidemiology', *American Journal of Epidemiology*, vol. 147, no. 3, pp. 222–9.
Dohrenwend, B.P. (2000) 'The role of adversity and stress in psychopathology: Some evidence and its implications for theory and research', *Journal of Health and Social Behaviour*, vol. 41, no. 1, pp. 1–19.
Dohrenwend, B.P. and Dohrenwend, B.S. (1982) 'Perspectives on the past and future of psychiatric epidemiology', *American Journal of Public Health*, vol. 72, pp. 1271–9.
Dohrenwend, B.P., Levan, I., Shrout, P., Shwartz, S., Naveh, G., Link B., Skodola, A. and Stueve, A. (1998) 'Ethnicity: socio-economic status and psychiatric disorders: a test of the social causation–social selection issue', in B.P. Dohrenwend (ed.) *Adversity, Stress and Psychopathology* (Oxford: Oxford University Press).
Dooley, D., Prause, J. and Ham-Rowbottom, K.A. (2000) 'Underemployment and depression: longitudinal relationships', *Journal of Health and Social Behavior*, vol. 41, pp. 421–36.
Dover, S. and McWilliam, C. (1992) 'Physical illness associated with depression in the elderly in community based and hospital patients', *Psychiatric Bulletin*, vol. 16, pp. 612–13.
Doyal, L. and Gough, I. (1991) *A Theory of Human Need* (London: Macmillan).
Drentea, P. (2000) 'Age, debt and anxiety', *Journal of Health and Social Behavior*, vol. 41, pp. 437–50.
Duncan, S. and Savage, M. (1989) 'Space, scale, locality', *ANTIPODE*, vol. 21, no. 3, pp. 179–207.
Dworkin, S.F. (1994) 'Somatization, distress and chronic pain', *Quality of Life Research*, vol. 3 (suppl 1), S77–S83.
Eaton, W. (1986) *The Sociology of Mental Disorders* (New York: Praeger).
Eaton, W.W. and Harrison, G. (2000) 'Epidemiology, social deprivation and community psychiatry', *Current Opinion in Psychiatry*, vol. 13, no. 2, pp. 185–7.
Edge, D. (2002) ' "Just dealing with it": Afro-Caribbean womens' perspectives on depression and managing adversity around childbirth', AUDGP North Conference presentation Kendal (January 2002).
Ehrenriech, B. and English, D. (1978) *For Her Own Good: 150 Years of Experts' Advice to Women* (New York: Anchor-Doubleday).
Eichenbaum, L. and Orbach, S. (1983) *Understanding Women: A Psychoanalytical Approach* (Harmondsworth: Penguin).

Elfkind, H.B. (1938) 'Is there an epidemiology of mental disease?', *American Journal of Public Health*, vol. 28, pp. 245–50.

Ellaway, A., Anderson, A. and Macintyre, S. (1997) 'Does area of residence affect body size and shape?', *International Journal of Obesity*, vol. 5. pp. 38–45.

Ellaway, A. and Macintyre, S. (1998) 'Does housing tenure predict health in the UK because it exposes people to different levels of housing related hazards in the home or its surroundings?', *Health and Place*, vol. 4, pp. 141–50.

Elliot, D.S., Wilson, W.J., Huzinga, D., Sampson, R.J., Elliot, A. and Rankin, B. (1996) 'The effects of neighbourhood disadvantage on adolescent development', *Journal of Research in Crime and Deliquency*, vol. 33, pp. 389–426.

Elliott, M. (2000) 'The stress process in its neighbourhood context', *Health and Place*, vol. 6, pp. 287–99.

Elstad, J.I. (1998) 'The psycho-social perspective on social inequalities in health', *Sociology Health and Illness*, vol. 20, no. 5, pp. 598–618.

Elton, P.J and Packer, J.M. (1986) 'A prospective randomised trial of the value of rehousing on the grounds of mental ill-health', *Journal of Chronic Disease*, vol. 39, pp. 221–7.

Engel, G. (1980) 'The biopsychosocial model', *American Journal of Psychiatry*, vol. 187, pp. 535–40.

Estroff, S. (1981) *Making it crazy: An Ethnography of Psychiatric clients in an American Community* (Berkeley: University of California Press).

Estroff, S.E. and Zimmer, C. (1994) 'Social networks, social support and violence among persons with severe persistent mental illness', in J. Monahan and H. Steadman (eds) *Violence and Mental Disorder: Developments in Risk Assessment* (Chicago: University of Chicago Press).

Eysenck, H.J. (1949) 'Training in clinical psychology: an English point of view', *American Psychologist*, vol. 4, pp. 173–6.

Eysenck, H.J. (1958) 'The psychiatric treatment of neurosis', Paper presented to the Royal Medico-Psychological Society, London.

Eysenck H.J. (1975) *The Future of Psychiatry* (London: Methuen).

Fabrega, H. and Manning, P.K. (1972) 'Disease, illness and deviant careers', in R.A. Scoot and J.D. Douglas (eds) *Theoretical Perspectives on Deviance* (New York: Basic Books).

Falloon, I. and Fadden, G. (1993) *Integrated Mental Health Care* (Cambridge: Cambridge University Press).

Falsetti, S.A., Resnick, H.S., Dansky, B.S., Lydiard, R.B. and Kilpatrick, D.G. (1995) 'The relationship of stress to panic disorder: cause or effect?', in C.M. Maxure (ed.) *Does Stress Cause Psychiatric Illness?* (Washington, DC: American Psychiatric Press).

Faris, R.E. and Dunham, H.W. (1939) *Mental Disorders in Urban Areas: An Ecological Study of Schizophrenia and Other Psychoses* (Chicago/London: University of Chicago Press).

Faulkner, A. (1997) *Knowing Our Own Minds* (London: Mental Health Foundation).

Fenton, S. and Sadiq-Sangster, A. (1996) 'Culture, relativism and mental distress', *Sociology of Health and Illness*, vol. 18, no. 1, pp. 66–85.

Fernando, S. (1988) *Race and Culture in Psychiatry* (Tavistock, Routledge).

Fernando, S. (1992) 'Psychiatry', *Open Mind*, vol. 58, pp. 8–9.

Finkelhor, D. (1979) *Sexually Victimized Children* (New York: Free Press).

Finn, S.E., Bailey, M., Schultz, R.T. and Faber, R. (1990) 'Subjective utility ratings of neuroleptics in treating schizophrenia', *Psychological Medicine*, vol. 20, pp. 843–8.

Firestone, R.W. (1997) *Suicide and the Inner Voice* (New York: Sage).

Fisher, N. and Baigent, B. (1996) 'Treatment with clozapine', *British Medical Journal*, vol. 313, p. 1262.

Forsythe, B. (1990) 'Mental and social diagnosis and the English Prison Commission 1914–1939', *Social Policy and Administration*, vol. 24, no. 3, pp. 237–53.

Foucault, M. (1965) *Madness and Civilisation* (New York: Random House).

Francis, E. (1988) 'Black people, dangerousness and psychiatric compulsion', in A. Brackx and C. Grimshaw (eds) *Mental Health Care in Crisis* (London: Pluto).

Freeling, P., Rao, B.M., Paykel, E.S., Sireling, L.I. and Burton, R.H. (1985) 'Unrecognised depression in general practice', *British Medical Journal*, vol. 290, pp. 1180–3.

Fryer, D. (1995) 'Labour market disadvantage, deprivation and mental health', *The Psychologist*, vol. 8, no. 6, pp. 265–72.

Fryers, T., Melzer, D. and Jenkins, R. (2001) *Mental Health Inequalities Report 1: A Systematic Literature Review* (Draft report to the Department of Health), Department of Public Health and Primary Care, University of Cambridge.

Gabe, J. and Bury, M. (1988) 'Tranquillisers as a social problem', *Sociological Review*, vol. 36, pp. 320–52.

Gabe, J. and Bury, M. (1991) 'Tranquillisers and the crises of health care', *Social Science and Medicine*, vol. 32, pp. 449–54.

Gabe, J. and Bury, M. (1996) 'Halcyon nights: a sociological account', *Sociology*, vol. 30, no. 2, pp. 447–71 (1991).

Gabe, J., Gustaffason, U. and Bury, M. (1991) 'Newspaper coverage of tranquiliser dependence', *Sociology of Health and Illness*, vol. 13, pp. 332–51.

Gabe, J., Kelleher, D. and Williams, G. (eds), (1994) *Challenging Medicine* (London: Routledge).

Gabe, J. and Thorogood, N. (1986) 'Prescribed drug use and the management of everyday life: the experiences of black and white working class women', *Sociological Review*, vol. 34, pp. 737–72.

Gabe, J. and Lipschitz-Phillips, S. (1984) 'Evil necessity? The meaning of benzodiazepine use for women patients from one general practice', *Sociology of Health and Illness*, vol. 4, no. 2, pp. 201–11.

Garfield, S.L. (1994) 'Outcome and process studies', in A.E. Bergin and S.L. Garfield (eds), *Handbook of Psychotherapy and Behavior Change* (New York: Wiley).

Gask, L., Lee, J., Donnan, S. and Roland, M. (2000) 'The impact of total purchasing and extended fund holding on mental health services: baseline aims and objectives of sites', *Journal of Mental Health*, vol. 9, no. 4, pp. 421–8.

Gask, L., Rogers, A., Roland, M. and Morris, D. (2000) *Improving Quality in Primary Care: A Practical Guide to the National Service Framework for Mental Health* (Manchester: NPCRDC).

Geddes, J., Freemantle, N., Harrison, P. and Bebbington, P. (2000) 'Atypical anti-psychotics in the treatment of schizophrenia: systematic overview and meta-regression analysis', *British Medical Journal*, vol. 321, pp. 1371–6.

Geil, R. (1998) 'Natural and human-made disasters', in B.P. Dohrenwend (ed.) *Adversity, Stress and Psychopathology* (New York: Oxford University Press).

Gesler, W.M. (1992) 'Therapeutic landscapes: medical issues in the light of the new cultural geography', *Social Science and Medicine*, vol. 34, no. 7, pp. 735–46.

Giggs, J.A. (1987) 'The spatial ecology of mental illness', in C. Smith and J. Giggs (eds) *Location and Stigma* (London: Unwin Hyman).

Gillam, S. and Miller, R. (1997) *A Public Health Experiment in Primary Care* (London: Kings Fund).

Gittens, D. (1998) *Madness In Its Place* (London: Routledge).

Glover, J. (1999) *Humanity: A Moral History of the Twentieth Century* (London: Jonathan Cape).

Goffman, E. (1961) *Asylums* (Harmondsworth: Penguin).

Goldberg, D. and Huxley, P. (1980) *Mental Illness in the Community* (London: Tavistock).

Goldberg, D. and Huxley, P. (1992) *Common Mental Disorders* (London: Routledge).

Goldie, N. (1978) 'The division of labour among mental health professions – a negotiated or an imposed order?', in M. Stacey and M. Reid (eds) *Health and the Division of Labour* (London: Croom Helm).

Goldsmith, H.F., Holzer, C.E. and Manderscheid, R.W. (1998) 'Neighborhood characteristics and mental illness', *Evaluation and Program Planning*, vol. 21, pp. 211–25.

Goldson, E. (1993) 'War is not good for children', in L.A. Leavitt and N.A. Fox (eds) *The Psychological Effects of War and Violence on Children* (Hillsdale, NJ: Erlbaum).

Gory, M.L., Ritchey, F.J., Ritchey, J. and Mullis, J. (1990) 'Depression among the homeless', *Journal of Health and Social Behaviour*, vol. 31, pp. 87–101.

Gottlieb, S. (2000) 'Rise in pre-school children receiving psychiatric drugs', *British Medical Journal*, vol. 320, p. 602.

Gottlieb, P., Cabrielson, G. and Kramp, P. (1987) 'Psychotic homicide in Copenhagen from 1959 to 1983', *Acta Psychiatrica Scandanavia*, vol. 76, pp. 285–92.

Gove, W. (1972) 'The relationship between sex roles, marital status and mental illness', *Social Forces*, vol. 51, pp. 33–44.

Gove, W. and Tudor, J.F. (1972) 'Adult sex roles and mental illness', *American Journal of Sociology*, vol. 78, pp. 812–35.

Graetz, B. (1993) 'Health consequences of unemployment and employment: longitudinal evidence for young men and women', *Social Science and Medicine*, vol. 36, pp. 715–24.

Graham, H. (2001) *Understanding Health Inequalities* (Buckingham: Open University Press).

Grant, C., Goodenough, T., Harvey, I. *et al.* (2000) 'A randomised controlled trial and economic evaluation of a referrals facilitator between primary care and the voluntary sector', *British Medical Journal*, vol. 320, pp. 419–23.

Grinker, R.G. (1975) 'The future educational needs of psychiatrists', *American Journal of Psychiatry*, vol. 132, no. 3, pp. 259–62.

Gutierrez-Lobos, K., Wolf, D., Scherer, M., Anderer, P. and Schmidl-Mohl, B. (2000) 'The gender gap in depression reconsidered: the influence of marital and employment status on the female/male ratio of treated incidence rates', *Social Psychiatry and Psychiatric Epidemiology*, vol. 35, pp. 201–2.

Guze, S.B. (1989) 'Biological psychiatry: is there any other kind?', *Psychological Medicine*, vol. 19, pp. 315–23.

Guze, S.B. and Helzer, J.B. (1985) 'The medical model and psychiatric disorders', in J. Cavenor (ed.) *Psychiatry* (Philadelphia: Lippincott).

Haley, J. (1963) *Strategies of Psychotherapy* (New York: Grune & Stratton).

Halpern, J.K.L., Sackett, P.R. and Binner, C.B. (1980) *The Myths of Deinstitutionalisation: Policies for the Mentally Disabled* (Boulder, CO: Westview).

Hambracht, M. and Hafner, H. (1996) 'Substance abuse and the onset of schizophrenia', *Biological Psychiatry*, vol. 40, pp. 1155–63.

Hamilton, M. (1973) 'Psychology in society: end or ends?', *Bulletin of the British Psychological Society*, vol. 26, pp. 185–9.

Harrison, G., Owens, D., Holton, A., Neilson, D. and Booth, D. (1988) 'A prospective study of severe mental disorder in Afro-Carribbean patients', *Psychological Medicine*, vol. 18, pp. 643–57.

Harrison, S. (1998) 'The politics of evidenced based medicine', *Policy and Politics*, vol. 26(1), pp. 15–31.

Haug, M. (1988) 'A re-examination of the hypothesis of de-professionalisation', *The Millbank Memorial Fund Quarterly*, vol. 66, no. 2, pp. 48–56.

Hawe, P. and Shiell, A. (2000) 'Social capital and health promotion: a review', *Social Science and Medicine*, vol. 51, p. 6.

Healy, D. (1997) *The Anti-Depressant Era* (London: Harvard University Press).

Healy, D. (2000) 'Sitting on it', *Open Mind*, vol. 102, pp. 18–19.

Helsing, K.J., Comstock, G.W. and Szklo, M. (1982) 'Causes of death in widowed populations', *American Journal of Epidemiology*, vol. 116, pp. 524–32.

Hemmenki, E. (1977) 'Polypharmacy among psychiatric patients', *Acta Psychiatrica Scandinavica*, vol. 56, pp. 347–56.

Henderson, C., Phelan, M., Loftus, L., Dall-Agnola, R. and Ruggeri, M. (1999) 'Comparison of patient satisfaction with community-based vs hospital psychiatric services', *Acta Psychiatrica Scandanavia*, vol. 99, pp. 188–95.

Hiday, V. (1995) 'The social context of mental illness and violence', *Journal of Health and Social Behaviour*, vol. 36, pp. 122–37.

Hiday, V. *et al.* (2001) 'Victimisation: a link between mental illness and violence', *International Journal of Law and Psychiatry*, vol. 24, pp. 559–72.

Hildebrand, P. (1982) 'Psychotherapy with older patients', *British Journal of Medical Psychology*, vol. 55, pp. 19–28.

HMSO (1992) *Report of the Committee of Inquiry into Complaints about Ashworth Hospital* (London: HMSO).

Hollingshead, A. and Redlich, R.C. (1958) *Social Class and Mental Illness* (New York: Wiley).

Hollon, S.D. and Beck, A.T. (1994) 'Cognitive and cognitive-behavioural therapies', in A.E. Bergin and S. Garfield (eds) *Handbook of Psychotherapy and Behavior Change* (London: Wiley).

Houghton, F. (2001) 'Does size matter?', Letter, *British Journal Psychiatry*, vol. 179, pp. 79–80.

Hubbert, F.A. and Whittington, J.E. (1993) 'Longtitudinal changes in mental state and personality measures', in B.D. Cox, F.A. Huppert and M.J. Whichelow (eds) *The Health and Lifestyle-Survey: Seven Years On* (Aldershot: Dartmouth).

Hutchenson, G. and Fahy, D. (2000) 'Profile of service users attending a voluntary mental health sector service', *Psychiatric Bulletin*, vol. 24, pp. 251–4.

Huxley, P., Rogers, A., Evans, S., Thomas, R., Robson, B., Gately, C. and Stordy, J. (2001) *Evaluating the impact of a locality based social policy intervention on mental health* (London: ESRC).

Hydle, I. (1993) 'Abuse and neglect in the elderly – a Nordic perspective', *Scandinavian Journal of Social Medicine*, vol. 21, no. 2, pp. 126–8.

Illich, I. (1975) *Medical Nemesis* (London: Marion Boyars).

Illich, I. (1977) *Limits to Medicine* (Harmondsworth: Penguin).

Ingleby, D. (1981) 'Understanding mental illness', in D. Ingleby (ed.) *Critical Psychiatry* (Harmondsworth: Penguin).

Jay, D.E. and Padilla, G.L. (1987) *Special Education Drop-Outs* (Menlo Park,CA: SRI).

Jenkins, R. (2001) 'Making psychiatric epidemiology useful: the contribution of epidemiology to government policy', *Acta Psychiatrica Scandnavica*, vol. 103, no. 10, pp. 2–14 Jan.

Jenkins, R., Lewis, G. and Bebbington, P. (1997) 'The National Psychiatric Morbidity Survey of Great Britain: initial findings from the household survey', *Psychological Medicine*, vol. 27, pp. 775–90.

Jenkins, R. and Singh, B. (2001) 'Mental disorder and disability in the population', in G. Thornicroft and G. Szmukler (eds) *Textbook of Community Psychiatry* (Oxford: Oxford University Press).

Jodelet, D. (1991) *Madness and Social Representation* (London: Harvester Wheatsheaf).

Johnson, J.G., Cohen, P., Dohrenwend, B.P., Link, B.G. and Brook, J.A. (1999) 'A longitudinal investigation of social causation and social selection processes involved in the association between socio-economic status and psychiatric disorders', *Journal of Abnormal Psychology*, vol. 108, pp. 490–9.

Jones, K. (1960) *Mental Health and Social Policy 1845–1959* (London: Routledge & Kegan Paul).

Joseph, K.S., Blais, L., Ernst, P. and Suissa, S. (1996) 'Increased morbidity and mortality related to asthma among asthmatic patients who use major tranquillisers', *British Medical Journal*, vol. 312, pp. 79–81.

Junginger, J. (1995) 'Command hallucinations and the prediction of dangerousness', *Psychiatric Services*, vol. 46, pp. 911–14.

Kadushin, C. (1969) *Why People Go To Psychiatrists* (New York: Atherton).

Kari, J., Donovan, D., Li, J. and Taylor, B. (1997) 'Adolescents' attitudes to primary care services in North London', *British Journal of General Practice*, vol. 47, pp. 109–10.

Karon, B.P. and VandenBos, G.R. (1981) *Psychotherapy of Schizophrenia: The Treatment of Choice* (New York: Jason Aronson).

Karp, D. (1994) 'Living with depression: illness and identity turning points', *Qualitative Health Research*, vol. 4, pp. 6–30.

Karp, D.A. (1994) *Speaking of Sadness: Depression, Disconnection and the Meanings of Illness* (New York: Oxford).

Kasl, S.V. and Harburg, E. (?) 'Mental health and the urban environment: some doubts and second thoughts', *Journal of Health and Social Behavior*, vol. 16, no. 3, pp. 268–80.

Kasl, S.V., Rodriguez, E. and Lasch, K.E. (1998) 'The impact of unemployment on health and well being', in B.P. Dohrenwend (ed.) *Adversity, Stress and Psychopathology* (Oxford: Oxford University Press).

Katz, R.C. and Watkins (1998) 'Adult victims of child sexual abuse', in A.S. Bellack and M. Hersen (eds), *Comprehensive Clinical Psychology*, vol. 9 (New York: Pergamon).

Kaufman, G.K., Jasinski, J.L. and Aldarando, E. (1994) 'Socio-cultural status and incidence of mental violence in Hispanic families', *Violence and Victims*, vol. 9, pp. 207–22.

Kawachi, I., Kennedy, B.P., Lochner, K. and Prothrow-Smith, D. (1997) 'Social capital, income inequality and mortality', *American Journal of Public Health*.

Kay, D., Beamish, P. and Roth, M. (1964) 'Old age disorders in Newcastle-upon-Tyne, Part 1: a study of prevalence', *British Journal of Psychiatry*, vol. 110, pp. 146–8.

Keane, T.M. (1998) 'Psychological effects of human combat', in B.P. Dohrenwend (ed.) *Adversity, Stress and Psychopathology* (Oxford: Oxford University Press).

Kellam, A.M.P. (1987) 'The neuroleptic syndrome so called: a review of the world literature', *British Journal of Psychiatry*, vol. 150, pp. 752–9.

Kelly, C.E. and Washafsky, L. (1987) 'Partner abuse in gay and lesbian couples', Paper presented at the 3rd National Family Violence Research Conference, Durham, New Hampshire.

Kelly, G. (1955) *The Psychology of Personal Constructs* (New York, Norton).

Kemker, S.S. and Khadivi, A. (1995) 'Psychiatric education: learning by assumption', in C.A. Ross and A. Pam (eds) *Pseudoscience in Biological Psychiatry: Blaming the Body* (New York: Wiley).

Kendler, K.S. (1998) 'Adversity, stress and psychopathology: a psychiatric genetic perspective', in B.P. Dohrenwend (ed.) *Adversity, Stress and Psychopathology* (Oxford: Oxford University Press).

Kernberg, O.F. (1973) 'Summary and conclusions of "Psychotherapy and psychoanalysis: final report of the Menninger Foundation's Psychotherapy Research Project"', *International Journal of Psychiatry*, vol. 11, pp. 62–77.

Kessler, R.C., House, J.S. and Turner, J.B. (1987) 'Unemployment and health in a community sample', *Journal of Health and Social Behaviour*, vol. 28, pp. 5–19.

Kessler, R.C., McGonagel, K.A., Zhai, S., Nelson, C.B., Hughes, M. and Eshleman, D. (1994) 'Lifetime and 12-month prevalence of DSM-III-R psychiatric disorders in the United States', *Archives of General Psychiatry*, vol. 51, pp. 8–19.

Kessler, R.C., Turner, J.B. and House, J.S. (1992) 'Intervening processes in the relationship between unemployment and health', *Psychological Medicine*, vol. 17, pp. 949–81.

Kitano, H.H.L. and Maki, M.T. (1996) 'Continuity, change and diversity: counseling Asian Americans', in P.B Pederson (ed.) *Counseling Across Cultures* (London: Sage).

Kitwood, T. (1988) 'The contribution of psychology to the understanding of senile dementia', in B. Gearing, M. Johnson and T. Heller (eds) *Mental Health Problems in Old Age* (London: Wiley).

Kitwood, T. (1997) *Dementia Reconsidered: The Person Comes First* (Buckingham: Open University Press).

Kitwood, T. and Bredin, K. (1992) 'Towards a theory of dementia care: personhood and well-being', *Ageing and Society*, vol. 10, pp. 177–96.

Kitzinger, C. (1993) 'Depoliticising the personal: a feminist slogan in feminist therapy', *Women's Studies International Forum*, vol. 16, no. 5, pp. 487–96.

Klass, A. (1975) *There's Gold in Them Thar Pills* (Harmondsworth: Penguin).

Kleinman, A. (1986) 'Some uses and misuses of the social sciences in medicine', in D.W. Fiske and R.A. Shweder (eds) *Metatheory and Social Science* (Chicago: Chicago University Press).

Kleinman, A. (1988) *Rethinking Psychiatry* (New York: Free Press).

Klerman, G.L. (1989) 'Psychiatric diagnostic categories: issues of validity and measurement, an invited comment on Mirowsky and Ross', *Journal of Health and Social Behavior*, vol. 30, pp. 26–30.

Klerman, G.L., Weissman, M.M., Markowitch, J., Glick, I., Wilner, P.H., Mason, B. and Shear, M.K. (1994) 'Medication and psychotherapy', in A.E. Bergin and S. Garfield (eds) *Handbook of Psychotherapy and Behavior Change* (London: Wiley).

Korten, A. and Henderson, S. (2000) 'The Australian National Survey of Mental Health and Well-Being. Common psychological symptoms and disablement', *British Journal of Psychiatry*, vol. 177, pp. 325–30.

Kreiger, N. (1994) 'Epidemiology and the web of causation: has anyone seen the spider?', *Social Science and Medicine*, vol. 39, pp. 887–903.

Kroll, J.K. (1988) *The Challenge of the Borderline Patient: Competency in Diagnosis and Treatment* (New York: Norton).

Kuller, L. (1999) 'Circular epidemiology', *American Journal of Epidemiology*, vol. 150, pp. 897–903.

Laing, R.D. and Esterson, A. (1964) *Sanity, Madness and the Family* (Harmondsworth: Penguin).

Lambert, M.J. and Bergin, A.E. (1994) 'The effectiveness of psychotherapy', in A.E. Bergin and S. Garfield (eds) *Handbook of Psychotherapy and Behavior Change* (London: Wiley).

Larkin, E.P., Murtagh, S. and Jones, S.J. (1988) 'A preliminary study of violent incidents in a Special Hospital (Rampton)', *British Journal of Psychiatry*, vol. 153, pp. 226–31.

Law, I. (1999) 'A discursive approach to therapy with men', in I. Parker (ed.) *Deconstructing Psychotherapy* (London: Sage).

Lawrence, M. and Maguire, M. (eds), (1997) *Psychotherapy with Women: Feminist Perspectives* (Basingstoke: Macmillan).

Lawson, A. (1989) 'A sociological and socio-anthropological perspective', in P. Williams, G. Wilkinson and K. Rawnsley (eds) *The Scope of Epidemiological Psychiatry* (London: Routledge).

Leff, J. (2001) *The Unbalanced Mind* (London: Faber).

Lelliot, P., Audini, B., Knapp, M. and Chisolm, D. (1996) 'The mental health residential care study: classification of facilities and description of residents', *British Journal of Psychiatry*, vol. 169, no. 2, pp. 139–47.

Lemert, E. (1967) *Human Deviance, Social Problems and Social Control* (Englewood Cliffs: Prentice-Hall).

Leon, D. and Walt, G. (eds) *Poverty, Inequality and Health* (Oxford: Oxford Medical Publications).

Levav, I. and Abrahamson, J.H. (1984) 'Emotional distress among concentration camp survivors: a community study in Jerusalem', *Psychological Medicine*, vol. 14, pp. 215–18.

Levav, I., Kahn, R. and Schwartz, S. (1998) 'The psychiatric after-effects of the holocaust on the second generation', *Psychological Medicine*, vol. 28, no. 4, pp. 775–80.

Levin, J. and McDevitt, J. (1993) *Hate Crimes: The Rising Tide of Bigotry and Bloodshed* (New York: Plenum).

Levin, J. and McDevitt, J. (1995) 'The research needed to understand hate crime', *The Chronicle of Higher Education*, vol. 41, B1–B2.

Levin, J.S. (1994) 'Religion and health: is there an association, is it valid and is it causal?', *Social Science and Medicine*, vol. 38, pp. 1475–82.

Lewis, G., Bebbington, P., Brugha, T., Farrell, M., Gill, B., Jenkins, R. and Meltzer, H. (1988) 'Socio-economic status, standard of living and neurotic disorder', *Lancet*, vol. 352, pp. 605–9.

Lewis, S. (1995) 'A search for meaning: making sense of depression', *Journal of Mental Health*, vol. 4, pp. 369–82.

Lidz, C.W., Mulvey, E.P. and Gardner, W. (1993) 'The accuracy of prediction of violence to others', *Journal of the American Medical Association*, vol. 269, pp. 1007–11.

Lie, G. and Gentlewarrior, S. (1991) 'Imtimate violence in lesbian relationships', Discussion of survey findings and practice implications, *Journal of Social Service Research*, vol. 15, pp. 41–59.

Light, D. (1985) 'Professional training and the future of psychiatry', in P. Brown (ed.) *Mental Health Care and Social Policy* (London: Routledge).

Lindow, V. (1994) *Self Help Alternatives to Mental Health Services* (London: MIND Publications).

Lindqvist, P. and Allebeck, P. (1989) 'Criminal homicide in North West Sweden 1970–1981. Alcohol intoxication, alcohol abuse and mental disease', *International Journal of Law and Psychiatry*, vol. 8, pp. 19–37.

Lindqvist, P. and Allebeck, P. (1990) 'Schizophrenia and crime: a longitudinal follow up of 644 schizophrenics in Stockholm', *British Journal of Psychiatry*, vol. 157, pp. 345–50.

Linehan, M. (1995) *Cognitive-Behavioural Therapy for Borderline Personality Disorder* (New York: Sage).

Link, B.G., Andrews, H.A. and Cullen, F.T. (1992) 'The violent and illegal behaviour of mental patients reconsidered', *American Sociological Review*, vol. 57, pp. 275–92.

Link, B., Bruce, G., Cullen, F.T., Struening, E., Shrout, P. and Dowhrenwend, B. (1989) 'A modified labelling theory approach to mental disorders: an empirical assessment', *American Sociological Review*, vol. 54, pp. 400–23.

Link, B.G., Susser, E., Stueve, A., Phelan, J., Moore, R., Struening, E. and Collen, M.E. (1994) 'Lifetime and five-year prevalence of homelessness in the United States', *American Journal of Public Health*, vol. 84, pp. 1907–12.

Littlejohns, P., Cluzeaut, F., Bale, R., Grismshaw, J., Feder, G. and Moran, S. (1999) 'The quantity and quality of clinical practice guidelines for the management of depression in primary care in the UK', *British Journal of General Practice*, vol. 49, pp. 205–10.

Littlewood, R. and Lipsedge, M. (1995) *Alliens and Alienists* (3rd edn) (Harmondsworth: Penguin).

Lomas, J. (1998) 'Social capital and health: implications for public health and epidemiology', *Social Science and Medicine*, vol. 47, no. 9, pp. 1181–8.

Lowenthal, M. (1965) 'Antecedents of isolation and mental illness in old age', *Archives of General Psychiatry*, vol. 12, pp. 245–54.

Lubin, B., Hornstra, R.K., Lewis, R.V. and Bechtel, B.S. (1973) 'Correlates of initial treatment assignment in a community mental health center', *Archives of General Psychiatry*, vol. 29, pp. 497–504.

Luhmann, N. (1982) *The Differentiation of Society* (New York: Columbia University Press).

Lyons, M. (1996) 'C. Wright Mills meets Prozac: the relevance of "social emotion" to the sociology of health and illness', in V. James and J. Gabe (eds) *Health and the Sociology of Emotions, Sociology of Health and Illness Monograph*, pp. 55–78.

Maas, S. (1998) 'Interventions at the worksite: from disease prevention to theory-based health promotion', Paper presented to the 12th Conference of the European Health Psychology Society: Prevention and Intervention, Vienna.

Maciejewski, P.K., Prigerson, H.G. and Mazure, C.M. (2001) 'Sex differences in event-related risk for major depression', *Psychological Medicine*, vol. 31, pp. 593–604.

McGorry, P., Curry, C. and Elkins, K. (1997) 'Psychosocial interventions in mental health disorders: developing evidence-based practice', *Current Opinion in Psychiatry*, vol. 10, no. 2, pp. 173–7.

Macintyre, S. (2000) 'Inequalities in health: is research gender blind', in D. Leon and G. Walt (eds) *Poverty, Inequality and Health* (Oxford: Oxford Medical Publications).

Macintyre, S. *et al.* (1993) 'Housing tenure and care access', *Journal of Epidemiology and Country Health*, vol. 55, no. 5, pp. 330–1.

McIntyre, S., MacIver, S. and Soomans, A. (1993) 'Area, class and health: should we be focusing on places or people?', *Journal of Social Policy*, vol. 22, no. 2, pp. 213–34.

McLeod, J.D. and Nonnemaker, J.M. (2000) 'Poverty and child emotional and behavioural problems: racial/ethnic differences in processes and effects', *Journal of Health and Social Behaviour*, vol. 41, pp. 137–61.

McNiel, D., Binder, R. and Greenfield, T. (1988) 'Predictions of violence in civily commited acute psychiatric patients', *American Journal of Psychiatry*, vol. 145, pp. 965–70.

Mann, A.H., Graham, N. and Ashby, D. (1984) 'Psychiatric illness in residential homes for the elderly: a survey in one London Borough', *Age and Ageing*, vol. 113, pp. 257–65.

Mann, B.J., Borduin, C.M., Hengeller, S.W. and Blaske, D.M. (1990) 'An investigation of systemic conceptualisations of parent child coalitions and symptom change', *Journal of Consulting and Clinical Psychology*, vol. 58, pp. 336–44.

Manor, O., Matthews, S. and Power, C. (1997) 'Comparing measures of health inequality', *Social Science and Medicine*, vol. 45, pp. 761–71.

Margolin, L. (1992) 'Sexual abuse by grandparents', *Child and Abuse and Neglect*, vol. 16, pp. 143–6.

Marshall, R. (1990) 'The genetics of schizophrenia: axiom or hypothesis?', in R.P. Bentall (ed.) *Reconstructing Schizophrenia* (London: Routledge).

Martin, J.P. (1985) *Hospitals in Trouble* (Oxford: Blackwell).

Masson, J. (1988) *Against Therapy* (London: HarperCollins).

Maule, M., Milen, J. and Williamson, J. (1984) 'Mental illness and physical health in older people', *Age and Ageing*, vol. 13, pp. 349–56.

May, C., and Mead, N., (1999) 'Patient-centredness: a history', in C. Dowrick and L. Frith (eds) *Ethical Problems in General Practice* (London: Routledge).

Mead, N., Bower, P. and Gask, L. (1997) 'Emotional problems in primary care: what is the potential for increasing the role of nurses?', *Journal of Advanced Nursing*, vol. 314, pp. 1337–41.

Mennen, F. (1993) 'Evaluation of risk factors in childhood sexual abuse', *Journal of the American Academy of Child and Adolescent Psychiatry*, vol. 32, pp. 934–9.

Miech, R.A., Caspi, A., Moffitt, T.E., Wright, B.R.E. and Silva, P.A. (1999) 'Low socio-economic status and mental disorders: A longitudinal study of selection and causation during young adulthood', *American Journal of Sociology*, vol. 104, no. 4, pp. 1096–131.

Meyer, A. (1952) *The Collected Papers of Adolph Meyer* (Baltimore: Johns Hopkins University Press).

Meyer, I.H. (1995) 'Minority stress and mental health in gay men', *Journal of Health and Social Behavior*, vol. 36, pp. 38–56.

Miller, N.E. and Magruder, K.M. (1999) *Cost-Effectiveness of Psychotherapy* (New York: Oxford University Press).

Mirowsky, J. and Reynolds, J.R. (2000) 'Age, depression and attrition in the national survey of families and households', *Sociological Methods and Research*, vol. 28, pp. 476–504.

Mirowsky, J. and Ross, C.E. (1984) 'Mexican culture and its emotional contradictions', *Journal of Health and Social Behaviour*, vol. 25, no. 1, pp. 213–34.

Mishara, A.L. (1994) 'A phenomenological critique of commonsensical assumptions in DSM-III-R: the avoidance of the patient's subjectivity', in J.Z. Sadler, O.P. Wiggins and M.A. Schwartz (eds) *Philosophical Perspectives on Psychiatric Diagnostic Classification* (Baltimore and London: Johns Hopkins University Press).

Mitchell, J. (1974) *Psychoanalysis and Feminism* (Harmondsworth: Penguin).

Mollica, R.F. Donelan, K., Tor, S. *et al.* (1993) 'The effect of trauma and confinement on functional health and mental health status of Cambodians living in Thailand-Cambodia border camps', *Journal of the American Medical Association*, vol. 270, pp. 581–6.

Monahan, J. (1993) 'Mental disorder and violence: another look', in S. Hodgins (ed.) *Mental Disorder and Crime* (New York: Sage).

Monahan, J. (2000) 'Clinical and actuarial predictions of violence', in D. Faigman *et al.* (eds) *Modern Scientific Evidence: The Law and Expert Testimony* (St Paul, NM: West Publishing Company).

Monahan, J. and Steadman, H.J. (1983) 'Crime and mental disorder: an epidemiological approach', in M. Tonry and N. Morris (eds) *Crime and Justice: An Annual Review of Research* (Chicago: Chicago University Press).

Monahan, J. and Steadman, H.J. (1994) 'Toward a rejuvenation of risk assessment research', in J. Monahan and H.J. Steadman (eds) *Violence and Mental Disorder: Developments in Risk Assessment* (Chicago: Chicago University Press).

Moncrieff, J. (2002) *Drugs in Modern Psychiatry: A History of Misrepresentation*, Animal Conference of Critical Psychiatry Network, Birmingham.

Monroe, S., Simons, A. and Thase, M. (1991) 'Onset of depression and time of treatment entry: roles of life stress', *Journal of Consulting and Clinical Psychology*, vol. 59, no. 4, pp. 566–73.

Morgan, K. and Gilleard, C. (1981) 'Patterns of hypnotic prescribing and usage in residential home for the elderly', *Neuropharmacology Journal*, vol. 20, pp. 1355–6.

Morse, B.J. (1995) 'Beyond the conflict tactics scale: assessing gender differences in partner violence', *Violence and Victims*, vol. 10, pp. 251–72.

Mortimer, P., Sammons, P., Stoll, L., Lewis, D. and Ecob, R. (1988) *School Matters: The Junior Years* (Wells: Open Books).

Mowbray, C.T., Moxley, D.P., Jasperr, C.A. and Howell, L.L. (1997) (eds) *Consumers as Providers in Psychiatric Rehabilitation* (Columbia: International Association of Psychosocial Rehabilitation Services).

Mumford, D.B., Minhas, F.A., Akhtar, S. and Mubbasher, M.H. (2000) 'Stress and psychiatric disorder in Rawalpindi. Community survey', *British Journal of Psychiatry*, vol. 177, pp. 557–62.

Muntaner, C., Eaton, W.W. and Chamberlain, C.D. (2000) 'Social inequalities in mental health: a review of concepts and underlying assumptions', *Health*, vol. 4, no. 1, pp. 89–109.

Muntaner, C., Eaton, W.W., Diala, C., Kessler, R.C. and Sorlie, P.D. (1998) 'Social class, assets, organisational control and the prevalence of common groups of psychiatric disorders', *Social Science and Medicine*, vol. 47, pp. 2043–53.

Muntaner, C., Wolyniec, P., McGrath, J. and Pulver, A.E. (1998) 'Arrest among psychotic inpatients; assessing the relationship to diagnosis, gender, number of admissions, and social class', *Social Psychiatry and Psychiatric Epidemiology*, vol. 33, pp. 274–82.

Murphy, E. (1982) 'Social origins of depression in old age', *British Journal of Psychiatry*, vol. 141, pp. 135–42.

Murphy, H.B.M. (1982) *Comparative Psychiatry: The International and Intercultural Distribution of Mental Illness* (Berlin: Springer Verlag).

Myers, J. and Bean, L. (1968) *A Decade Later: A Follow Up of Social Class and Mental Illness* (New York: Wiley).

Nan, L., Dean, A. and Enzel, W. (1986) *Social Support, Life Events, and Depression* (Orlando, FL: Academic Press).

Nazroo, J. (1997) *Ethnicity and Mental Health* (London: Policy Studies Institute).

Nazroo, J. (1998) 'Rethinking the relationship between ethnicity and mental health: the British fourth National Survey of Ethnic Minorities', *Social Psychiatry and Psychiatric Epidemiology*, vol. 33, no. 4, pp. 145–8.

Nazroo, J., Edwards, A.C. and Brown, G.W. (1998) 'Gender differences in the prevalence of depression: artefact, alternative disorders, biology or roles?', *Sociology of Health and Illness*, vol. 20, no. 3, pp. 312–30.

Noble, P. and Rodger, S. (1989) 'Violence by psychiatric inpatients', *British Journal of Psychiatry*, vol. 155, pp. 384–90.

Noll, R. (1996) *The Jung Cult: Origins of a Charismatic Movement* (London: Fontana).

North, C.S., Thompson, S.J., Polio, D.E., Ricci, D.A. and Smith, E.M. (1997) 'A diagnostic comparison of homeless and non-homeless patients in an urban mental health clinic', *Social Psychiatry and Psychiatric Epidemiology*, vol. 32, no. 4, pp. 236–40.

O'Connor, R.C. and Sheehy, N.P. (2001) 'Suicidal behaviour', *The Psychologist*, vol. 14, no. 1, pp. 20–4.

O'Connor, R.C., Sheehy, N.P. and O'Connor, D.B. (1999) 'The classification of completed suicide into sub-types', *Journal of Mental Health*, vol. 8, pp. 629–37.

Odell, S.M. and Commander, M.J. (2000) 'Risk factors for homelessness among people with psychotic disorders', *Social Psychiatry and Psychiatric Epidemiology*, vol. 35, p. 9.

Olds, D., Henderson, C.R., Tatelbaum, R. and Chamberlin, R. (1988) 'Improving the life course development of socially disadvantaged mothers: a randomised trial of nurse home visitation', *American Journal of Public Health*, vol. 78, pp. 1436–45.

Olfson, M. and Pincus, H.A. (1999) 'Outpatient psychotherapy in the United States: the National Medical Expenditure Survey', in N.E. Miller and K.M. Magruder (eds) *Cost-Effectiveness of Psychotherapy* (New York: Oxford University Press).

Oliver, M. (1990) *The Politics of Disability* (Basingstoke: Macmillan).

Onyett, S., Heppleston, T. and Bushnell, D. (1994) 'A national survey of community mental health team structure and process', *Journal of Mental Health*, vol. 3, pp. 175–94.

Orbach, S. (1978) *Fat is a Feminist Issue* (London: Hamlyn).

Orbach, S. (1986) *Hunger Strike* (London: Faber).

Ostler, K., Thompson, C., Kinmoth, A.-L.K., Peveler, L., Stevens, L. and Stevens, A. (2001) 'Influence of socio-economic deprivation on the prevalence and outcome of depression in primary care: the Hampshire Depression Project', *British Journal of Psychiatry*, vol. 178, pp. 12–17.

Paivarinta, A., Verkoniemi, A., Nininsto, Kivela, S.-L. and Sulkava, R. (1999) 'The prevalence and associates of depressive disorders in the oldest-old Finns', *Social Psychiatry and Psychiatric Epidemiology*, vol. 34, pp. 352–9.

Parker, I., Georgaca, E., Harper, D., McLaughlin, T. and Stowell-Smith, M. (1997) *Deconstructing Psychopathology* (London: Sage).

Parkman, S., Davies, S., Leese, M., Phelan, M. and Thornicroft, G. (1997) 'Ethnic differences in satisfaction with mental health services among representative people with psychosis in South London: PriSM study 4', *British Journal of Psychiatry*, vol. 171, pp. 260–4.

Parr, H. (2000) 'Interpreting the "hidden social geographies" of mental health: ethnographies of inclusion and exclusion in semi-institutional places', *Health and Place*, vol. 6, no. 3, pp. 225–37.

Patel, V. (2001) 'Poverty, inequality and mental health in developing countries' in D. Leon and G. Walt (eds) *Poverty, Inequality and Health* (Oxford: Oxford Medical Publications).

Paveza, G.J., Cohen, J.G. and Esdorfer, C. (1992) 'Severe family violence and Alzheimer's Disease: prevalence and risk factors', *Gerontologist*, vol. 32, no. 4, pp. 493–7.

Paykel, E.S., Abbott, R., Jenkins, R., Brugha, T.S. and Meltzer, H. (2000) 'Urban-rural mental health differences in Great Britain: findings from the National Morbidity Survey', *Psychological Medicine*, vol. 30, no. 2, pp. 269–80.

Pearlin, L.I. (1975) 'Sex roles and depression', in N. Datan and L. Ginsberg (eds) *Lifespan Developmental Psychology* (New York: Academic Press).

Pearlin, L.I. (1989) 'The sociological study of stress', *Journal of Health and Social Behaviour*, vol. 30, no. 3, pp. 241–56.

Pearlin, L.I. and Skaff, M.M. (1996) 'Stress and the life course: a paradigmatic alliance', *The Gerontologist*, vol. 36, pp. 239–47.

Penfold, P.S. and Walker, G.A. (1984) *Women and the Psychiatric Paradox* (Milton Keynes: Open University Press).

Pescosolido, B., Gardner, B. and Lubell, K. (1998) 'How people get into mental health services: stories of choice, coercion and "muddling through" from "first timers"', *Social Science and Medicine*, vol. 46, no. 2, pp. 275–86.

Phillips, D. (1968) 'Social class and psychological disturbance: the influence of positive and negative experiences', *Social Psychiatry*, vol. 3, pp. 41–6.

Phillipson, C. (1989) 'Developing a political economy of drugs and older people', *Ageing and Society*, vol. 9, pp. 431–40.

Philo, C. (1997) 'Across the water: reviewing geographical studies of asylums and other mental health facilities', *Health and Place*, vol. 3, no. 2, pp. 73–89.

Piccinelli, M. and Wilkinson, G. (2000) 'Gender differences in depression', *The British Journal of Psychiatry*, vol. 177, pp. 486–92.

Pilger, J. (1989) *A Secret Country* (London: Vantage).

Pilgrim, D. (1997) *Psychotherapy and Society* (London: Sage).

Pilgrim, D. (2001) 'Disordered personalities and disordered concepts', *Journal of Mental Health*, vol. 10, no. 3, pp. 253–66.

Pilgrim, D. and Bentall, R.P. (1999) 'The medicalisation of misery: a critical realist analysis of the concept of depression', *Journal of Mental Health*, vol. 8, no. 3), pp. 261–74.

Pilgrim, D. and Guinan, P. (1999) 'Rethinking the evidence about therapist sexual abuse', *European Journal of Psychology, Counselling and Psychotherapy*, vol. 29, no. 1), pp. 50–61.

Pilgrim, D. and Rogers, A. (1994) ' "Something old, something new" . . . sociology and the organisation of psychiatry', *Sociology*, vol. 28, no. 2, pp. 521–38.

Pilgrim, D. and Rogers, A. (1999) *A Sociology of Mental Health and Illness* (Buckingham: Open University Press).

Pilgrim, D., Rogers, A., Clarke, S. and Clark, W. (1997) 'Entering psychological treatment: decision-making factors for GPs and service users', *Journal of Interprofessional Care*, vol. 11, no. 3, pp. 313–23.

Pilgrim, D. and Treacher, A. (1992) *Clinical Psychology Observed* (London: Routledge).

Pilgrim, D. and Waldron, L. (1998) 'User involvement in mental health service development: how far can it go?', *Journal of Mental Health*, vol. 7, no. 1, pp. 95–104.

Pilkonis, P.A., Imber, S., Lewis, P. and Rubinsky, P. (1984) 'A comparative outcome study of individual, group and conjoint psychotherapy', *Archives of General Psychiatry*, vol. 41, pp. 431–7.

Pinfold, V. (2000) 'Building up safe havens . . . all around the world: users' experiences of living in the community with mental health problems', *Health and Place*, vol. 6, no. 3, pp. 201–12.

Pokorny, A.D. (1983) 'Prediction of suicide in psychiatric patients', Report of a prospective study, *Archives of General Psychiatry*, vol. 40, pp. 249–57.

Porter, B. and O'Leary, K.D. (1980) 'Marital discord and child behaviour problems', *Journal of Abnormal Child Psychology*, vol. 8, pp. 287–95.

Porter, R. (1989) *A Social History of Madness* (London: Routledge).

Portes, A. (1998) 'Social capital: its origins and applications in modern sociology', *Annual Review of Sociology*, vol. 24, pp. 1–24.

Power, L. and Pilgrim, D. (1990) 'The fee in psychotherapy: practitioners' accounts', *Counselling Psychology Quarterly*, vol. 3, no. 2, pp. 153–7.

Price, R.H., Van Ryn, M. and Vinokurl, A. (1992) 'Impact of preventative job search intervention on the likelihood of depression amongst the unemployed', *Journal of Health and Social Behavior*, vol. 33, pp. 158–67.

Priest, R.G., Vize, C., Roberts, A., Roberts, M. and Tylee A. (1996) 'Lay people's attitudes to treatment of depression: results of opinion poll for Defeat Depression Campaign just before its launch', *British Medical Journal*, vol. 313, pp. 858–9.

Prior, C., Clements, J. and Rowett, M. (2001) 'Users' experiences of treatments must be considered', *British Medical Journal*, vol. 322, p. 924.

Prior, L. (1991) 'Mind body and behaviour: theorisations of madness and the organisation of therapy', *Sociology*, vol. 25, no. 3, pp. 403–22.

Quinn, K.P. and Epstein, M.H. (1998) 'Characteristics of children, youth and families served by local interagency systems of care', in M.H. Epstein, K. Kutash and A. Duchnowski (eds) *Outcomes for Children and Youth with Behavioural and Emotional Disorders and their Families* (Austin: Pro-Ed).

Quirk, A. and Lelliott, P. (2001) 'What do we know about life on acute psychiatric wards in the UK?: a review of the research evidence', *Social Science and Medicine*, vol. 53, no. 192, pp. 1565–74.

Rabkin, J. (1979) 'Criminal behaviour of discharged psychiatric patients: a critical review of the research', *Psychological Bulletin*, vol. 86, pp. 1–27.

Raja, M., Azzoni, A. and Luhich, L. (1997) 'Aggressive and violent behaviour in a population of psychiatric inpatients', *Social Psychiatry and Psychiatric Epidemiology*, vol. 32, pp. 428–34.

Ramon, S. and Giannichedda, M.G (eds), (1988) *Psychiatry in Transition: The British and Italian Experience* (Cambridge: Polity Press).

Ranger, C. (1989) 'Race, culture and "cannabis psychosis": the role of social factors in the construction of a disease category', *New Community*, vol. 15, no. 3, pp. 357–69.

Raviv, A., Sills, R., Raviv, A. and Wilansky, P. (2000) 'Adolescents' help-seeking behaviour: the difference between self and other referral', *Journal of Adolescence*, vol. 23, no. 6, pp. 721–40.

Regier, D., Boyd, J., Burke, *et al.* (1988) 'Prevalence of mental disorders in the United States', *Archives of General Psychiatry*, vol. 45, pp. 977–85.

Regier, D.A., Farmer, M.E., Raue, D.A. *et al.* (1990) 'Comorbidity of mental disorders with alcohol and other drug abuse: results from the epidemiologic catchment area (ECA) study', *Journal of the American Medical Association*, vol. 264, pp. 2511–18.

Robertson, A. (1998) 'Critical reflections on the politics of need: implications for public policy', *Social Science and Medicine*, vol. 47, no. 10, pp. 1419–30.

Robins, L.N. and Reiger, D.A. (eds), (1991) *Psychiatric Disorders in America: The Epidemiologic Catchment Area Study* (New York: Free Press).

Rogers, A. (1990) 'Policing mental disorder: Controversies, myths and realities', *Social Policy and Administration*, vol. 24, no. 3, pp. 226–7.

Rogers, A., Campbell, S., Gask, L., Marshall, M., Haliwell, S. and Pickard, S. (2002) 'Some National Service Frameworks are more equal than other: implementing clinical governance for mental health in primary care groups and trusts', *Journal of Mental Health*, vol. 11, no. 2, pp. 199–212.

Rogers, A., Day, J., Williams, B. *et al.* (1998) 'The meaning and management of medication: perspectives of patients with a diagnosis of schizophrenia', *Social Science and Medicine*, vol. 47, no. 9, pp. 1313–23.

Rogers, A., May, C. and Oliver, D. (2001) 'Experiencing depression; experiencing the depressed: the separate worlds of patients and doctors', *Journal of Mental Health*, vol. 10, no. 3, pp. 317–33.

Rogers, A., Hassell, K., Nicolass, G. (1999) *Demanding Patients?: Analysing the Use of Primary Care* (Buckingham: Open University Press).

Rogers, A. and Pilgrim, D. (1986) 'Mental Health reforms: some contrasts between Britain and Italy', *Free Associations*, vol. 6, pp. 65–80.

Rogers, A. and Pilgrim, D. (1991) ' "Pulling down churches": accounting for the British mental health users' movement', *Sociology of Health and Illness*, vol. 13, no. 2, pp. 129–48.

Rogers, A. and Pilgrim, D. (1993) 'Service users views of psychiatric treatment', *Sociology of Health and Illness*, vol. 15, no. 5, pp. 612–31.

Rogers, A. and Pilgrim, D. (1997) 'The contribution of lay knowledge to the understanding and promotion of mental health', *Journal of Mental Health*, vol. 6, no. 1, pp. 23–35.

Rogers, A. and Pilgrim, D. (2001) *Mental Health and Policy in Britain* (2nd edn) (Basingstoke: Palgrave).

Rogers, A., Pilgrim, D. and Lacey, R. (1993) *Experiencing Psychiatry: User's Views of Services* (Basingstoke: Macmillan).

Romme, M. and Escher, S. (1993) *Accepting Voices* (London: MIND Publications).

Rose, N. (1990) *Governing the Soul* (London: Routledge).

Rose, S., Kamin, L.T. and Lewontin, R.C. (1984) *Not in Our Genes* (Harmondsworth: Penguin).

Rosen, G. (1979) *Madness In Society* (New York: Harper).

Rosenfeld, S. (1999) 'Gender and Mental Health: Do women have more psychopathology, men more or both the same?', in A. Horwitz and T. Scheid (eds) *A Handbook for the Study of Mental Health* (Cambridge: Cambridge University Press).

Rosenhan, D.L. (1973), 'On being sane in insane places', *Science*, vol. 179, pp. 250–8.

Ross, C., Mirowsky, J. and Pribesh, S. (2001) 'Powerlessness and the amplification of threat: neighbourhood disadvantage, disorder and mistrust', *American Sociological Review*, vol. 66, pp. 568–91.

Ross, C.A. and Pam, A. (eds) (1995) *Pseudoscience in Biological Psychiatry: Blaming the Body* (New York: Wiley).

Ross, C.E. (2000) 'Neighbourhood disadvantage and adult depression', *Journal of Health and Social Behavior*, vol. 41, pp. 177–87.

Roth, M. (1973) 'Psychiatry and its critics', *British Journal of Psychiatry*, vol. 122, p. 374.

Royal College of Psychiatrists (1996) *Report on the Use of Electro-Convulsive Therapy* (London: Royal College of Psychiatrists).

Rudin, M., Zalewski, and Boomer-Turner, J. (1995) 'Characteristics of child abuse victims according to perpetrator gender', *Child Abuse and Neglect*, vol. 19, pp. 963–73.

Russell, D. (1983) 'The incidence and prevalence of intrafamilial and extrafamilial sexual abuse of female children', *Child Abuse and Neglect*, vol. 7, pp. 133–46.

Russell, D. (1995) *Women, Madness and Medicine* (Oxford: Polity).

Rutter, M., Maughan, B., Mortimore, P., Ouston, J. and Smith, A. (1979) *Fifteen Thousand Hours: Secondary Schools and their Effects on Children* (Cambridge, MA: Harvard University Press).

Ryan, W. (ed.) (1969) *Distress in the City: Essays on the Design and Administration of Urban Mental Health Services* (Cleveland: Case Western Reserve University Press).

SCPR (1999) *Health Survey for England 1994–96* (London: Department of Health).

Sacker, A., School, I. and Bartley, M. (1999) 'Childhood influences on socio-economic inequalities in adult mental health: path analysis as an aid to understanding', *Health Variations*, vol. 4, pp. 8–10 (Lancaster: ESRC).

Sackheim, D.K. and Devine, S.E. (1995) 'Trauma-related syndromes', in C.A. Ross and A. Pam (eds) *Pseudo-Science in Biological Psychiatry: Blaming the Body* (New York: Wiley).

Saks, M. (1983) 'Removing the blinkers? A recent contribution to the sociology of the professions', *The Sociological Review*, vol. 33, pp. 1–21.

Sainsbury Centre (1998) *Acute Problems: A Survey of the Quality of Care in Acute Psychiatric Wards* (London: Sainsbury Centre for Mental Health).

Salzman, C., Shader, R., Scott, D. and Binstock, W. (1970) 'Interviewer anger and patient dropout in walk-in clinics', *Comprehensive Psychiatry*, vol. 11, pp. 267–73.

Sampson, R.J. (1988) 'Local friendship ties and community attachment', *American Sociological Review*, vol. 53, pp. 766–79.

Sampson, R.J., Raudenbush, S.W. and Earles, F. (1997) 'Neighbourhoods and violent crime: a multilevel study of collective efficacy', *Science*, vol. 277, pp. 918–24.

Samson, C. (1995) 'The fracturing of medical dominance in British psychiatry', *Sociology of Health and Illness*, vol. 17, no. 2, pp. 245–68.

Samuels, A. (1998) *The Political Psyche* (London: Routledge).

Satlin, A., Liptzin, B., Jenike, M., Salzman, C. and Pinals, S. (1999) 'The elderly person', in A.M. Nicholi (ed.) *The Harvard Guide to Psychiatry* (London: Harvard University Press).

Saunders, S.M., Resnick, M.D., Hoberman, H.M. and Blum, R.W. (1994) 'Formal help-seeking behaviour of adolescents identifying themselves as having mental health problems', *Journal of the American Academy of Child and Adolescent Psychiatry*, vol. 33, pp. 718–28.

Savio, M. and Righetti, A. (1993) 'Co-operatives as a social enterprise in Italy: a place for social integration and rehabilitation', *Acta Psychiatrica Scandinavia*, vol. 88, pp. 238–42.

Sayce, L. (2000) *From Psychiatric Patient to Citizen: Overcoming Discrimination and Social Exclusion* (Basingstoke: Macmillan).

Scheff, T. (1966) *Being Mentally Ill: A Sociological Theory* (Chicago: Aldine).

Schieman, S., van Gundy, K. and Taylor, J. (2001) 'Status, role, and resource explanations for age patterns in psychological distress', *Journal of Health and Social Behavior*, vol. 42, pp. 80–96.

Schwabe, A.M. and Kodras, J. (2000) 'Race, class and psychological distress: contextual variations across four American communities', *Health*, vol. 4, no. 2, pp. 234–60.

Scull, A. (1979) *Museums of Madness* (Harmondsworth: Penguin).

Segal, S., Baumohl, J. and Moyles, E. (1980) 'Neighbourhood types and community reaction to the mentally ill: a paradox of intensity', *Journal of Health and Social Behaviour*, vo. 21, no. 4, pp. 345–59.

Segal, S.P., Cohen, D., Marder, S.P. (1992) 'Neuroleptic medication and prescription practices with sheltered care residents – a 12 year perspective', *American Journal of Public Health*, vol. 82, no. 6, pp. 846–52.

Seigrist, J. (2000) 'Place, social exchange and health: a proposed sociological framework', *Social Science and Medicine*, vol. 51, no. 9, pp. 1283–93.

Sennett, R. and Cobb, J. (1980) *The Hidden Injuries of Class* (London: Faber & Faber).

Sereny, G. (1995) *Albert Speer: His Battle for Truth* (London: Macmillan).

Shepperd, G., Beadsmoore, A., and Moore, C. (1997) 'Relation between bed use, social deprivation and overall bed availability in acute adult psychiatric units and alternative residential options: a cross sectional survey, one day census data and staff interviews', *British Medical Journal*, vol. 314, no. 7076, pp. 262–6.

Shorter, E. (1997) *A History of Psychiatry: From the Era of the Asylum to the Age of Prozac* (Chichester: Wiley).

Showalter, E. (1987) *The Female Malady: Women Madness and English Culture 1830–1980* (London: Virago).

Silver, E. (2000) 'Race, neighbourhood, disadvantage, and violence among persons with mental disorders: the importance of contextual measurement', *Law and Human Behavior*, vol. 24, pp. 449–56.

Silver, E., Mulvey, E. and Monahan, J. (1999) 'Assessing violence risk among discharged psychiatric patients: towards an ecological approach', *Law and Human Behaviour*, vol. 23, no. 2, pp. 237–47.

Slater, P. (1977) *Origins and Significance of the Frankfurt School* (London: Routledge).

Sloane, R.B., Staples, F.R., Cristol, A.H., Yorkston, N.J. and Whipple, K. (1975) *Psychotherapy versus Behavior Therapy*, (Cambridge, MA: Harvard University Press).

Smith, C.J. (1987) 'Mental health and the fiscal crisis: the prospects for a socially conscious urban geography', *Urban Geography*, vol. 10, pp. 186–95.

Smith, C.J. and Giggs, J.A. (eds) (1988) *Location and Stigma: Contemporary Perspectives on Mental Health and Mental Health Care* (London: Unwin Hyman).

Smith D.M. (1984) 'Geographical approaches to mental health', in H.L. Freeman (ed.) *Mental Health and the Environment* (London: Churchill Livingstone).

Snowden, J. and Donnelly, M. (1986) 'A study of depression in nursing homes', *Journal of Psychiatric Research*, vol. 20, pp. 327–33.

Solkoff, N. (1992) 'Children of survivors of the holocaust. A critical review of the literature', *American Journal of Orthopsyhiatry*, vol. 62, pp. 342–58.

South, S.J. and Crowder, K.D. (1997) 'Escaping distressed neighbourhoods: individual, community, and metropolitan influences', *American Journal of Sociology*, vol. 102, pp. 1040–84.

Soyka, M. (2000) 'Substance misuse, psychiatric disorder and violent and disturbed behaviour', *British Journal of Psychiatry*, vol. 176, pp. 345–50.

Spagnoli, A., Forest, G., MacDonald, A. and Williams, P. (1986) 'Dementia and depression in Italian geriatric institutions', *International Journal of Geriatric Psychiatry*, vol. 1, pp. 15–23.

Spector, R. (2001) 'Is there racial bias in clinicians' perceptions of the dangerousness of psychiatric patients? A review of the literature', *Journal of Mental Health*, vol. 10, no. 1, pp. 5–16.

Srole, L. and Langer, T.S. (1962) *Mental Health in the Metropolis: The Midtown Manhattan Study* (New York: McGraw Hill).

Stansfeld, S.A., Head, J. and Marmot, M.G. (1998) 'Explaining social class differences in depression and well being', *Social Psychiatry and Psychiatric Epidemiology*, vol. 33, pp. 1–9.

Steadman, H.J., Mulvey, E.P., Monahan, J., Robbins, P.C., Applebaum, P.S., Grisso, T., Roth, L.H. and Silver, E. (1998) 'Violence by people discharged from acute psychiatric inpatient facilities and by others in the same neighbourhood', *Archives of General Psychiatry*, vol. 55, pp. 1–9.

Stolberg, A.L., Mullett, E. and Gourley, E.V. (1998) 'Families of divorce', in A.S. Bellack and M. Hersen (eds) *Comprehensive Clinical Psychology*, vol. 9 (New York: Pergamon).

Stone, M. (1985) 'Shellshock and the psychologists', in W.F. Bynum, R. Porter and M. Shepherd (eds) *The Anatomy of Madness*, vol. 2 (London: Tavistock).

Straus, M.A. (1993) 'Physical assaults by wives: a major social problem', in R.J. Gelles and D. Loseke (eds) *Current Controversies on Family Violence* (Newbury Park: Sage).

Straus, M.A. and Gelles, R.J. (1990) *Physical Violence in American Families: Risk Factors and Adaptations to Violence in 8,145 families* (New Brunswick: Transaction Publishers).

Stueve, A. and Link, B.G. (1997) 'Violence and psychiatric disorders: result, from an epidemiological study of young adults in Israel', *Psychiatric Quarterly*, vol. 68, pp. 327–42.

Stueve, A. and Link, B.G. (1998) 'Gender differences in the relationship between mental illness and violence: evidence from a community-based epidemiological study in Israel', *Social Psychiatry and Psychiatric Epidemiology*, vol. 33, pp. S61–S67.

Sue, S., Fujino, D.C., Hu, L.T., Takeuchi, D.T. and Zane, N.W.S. (1991) 'Community mental health services for ethnic minority groups', *Journal of Counseling Psychology*, vol. 59, pp. 533–40.

Sullivan, G., Burnham, A. and Koegel, P. (2000) 'Pathways to homelessness among the mentally ill', *Social Psychiatry and Psychiatric Epidemiology*, vol. 35, pp. 444–50.

Swan, V. (1999) 'Narrative, Foucault and feminism: implications for therapeutic practice', in I. Parker (ed.) *Deconstructing Psychotherapy* (London: Sage).

Swanson, J. *et al.* (1990) 'Violence and psychiatric disorder in the community: evidence from the epidemiological catchment area surveys', *Hospital and Community Psychiatry*, vol. 41, pp. 761–70.

Swartz, M.S., Swanson, J.W., Hiday, V.A., Borum, W., Wagner, R. and Burns, B.J. (1998) 'Taking the wrong drugs: the role of substance abuse and medication non-compliance in violence among severely mentally ill individuals', *Social Psychiatry and Psychiatric Epidemiology*, vol. 33, pp. S75–S80.

Szasz T.S. (1961) 'The uses of naming and the origin of the myth of mental illness', *American Psychologist*, vol. 16, pp. 59–65.

Szasz, T.S. (1963) *Law Liberty and Psychiatry* (New York: Macmillan).

Tardiff, K. and Sweillam, A. (1982) 'Assault, suicide and mental illness', *American Journal of Psychiatry*, vol. 37, pp. 164–9.

Tarrier, N., Beckett, R., Harwood, S., Baker, A., Yusupoff, L. and Ugarteburn, I. (1993) 'A trial of two cognitive-behavioural methods of treating drug-resistant residual psychotic symptoms in schizophrenic patients', *British Journal of Psychiatry*, vol. 162, pp. 524–32.

Taylor, P.J. (1985) 'Motives for offending among violent psychotic men', *British Journal of Psychiatry*, vol. 147, pp. 491–8.

Teeson, M., Hodder, T. and Buhrich, N. (2000) 'Substance use disorders among homeless people in inner Sydney', *Social Psychiatry and Psychiatric Epidemiology*, vol. 35, no. 10, pp. 451–6.

Telles, B. and Pollack, M. (1981) 'Feeling sick: the experience and legitimation of illness', *Social Science and Medicine*, vol. 15, no. 9, pp. 243–51.

Tennov, D. (1976) *Psychotherapy: The Hazardous Cure* (New York: Anchor).

Teplin, L. (1990) 'The prevalence of severe mental disorder among male urban jail detainees: comparison with the Epidemiologic Catchment Area program', *American Journal of Public Health*, vol. 30, pp. 663–9.

Tesh, S. (1990) *Hidden Arguments: Political Ideology and Disease Prevention Policy* (New Brunswick: Rutgers University Press).

Thoits, P.A. (1995) 'Stress, coping and social support processes – where we are and what next', *Journal of Health and Social Behaviour* (Extra issue) pp. 53–79.

Thomas, P. and Romme, M. (1997) 'Psychiatry and the politics of the underclass', *British Journal of Psychiatry*, vol. 170, pp. 192ff.

Thomas, R., Evans, S., Gately C., Stordy, J., Huxley, P., Rogers, A. and Robson, B. (2002) 'State-event relations among indicators of susceptibility to mental distress in Wythenshawe', *Social Science and Medicine*, pp. 921–35

Tjaden, P. and Thoennes, R. (1998) *The National Violence Against Women Survey* (Washington: US Congress).

Tkatchenko, E., McKee, M., Tsouros, A.D. (2000) 'Public health in Russia: the view from the inside', *Health Policy Planning*, vol. 15, no. 2, pp. 164–9.

Toro, P.A. (1998) 'Homelessness', in A.S. Bellack and M. Hersen (eds) *Comprehensive Clinical Psychology*, vol. 9 (New York: Pergamon).

Trethowan, W.H. (1977) *The Role of Psychologists in the Health Service* (London: HMSO).

Tudor-Hart, J. (1971) 'The inverse care law', *The Lancet*, pp. 405–12.

Turner, B.S. (1986) *Equality* (London: Tavistock).

Tyrer, P. (1999) 'The national service framework: a scaffold for mental health', *British Medical Journal*, vol. 319, pp. 1017–18.

United States Congress (1992) H.R. 4797 102d Congress 2nd Session.

Ussher, J. (1991) *Women's Madness: Misogyny or Mental Illness?* (London: Harvester-Wheatsheaf).

Ussher, J.M. and Nicolson, P. (eds) (1992) *Gender Issues in Clinical Psychology* (London: Routledge).

van Praag, H.M. (1977) 'The significance of dopamine for the mode of action of neuroleptics and pathogenesis of schizophrenia', *British Journal of Psychiatry*, vol. 130, pp. 463–74.

Van Putten, T. (1975) 'The many faces of akathisia', *Comprehensive Psychiatry*, vol. 16, pp. 43–7.

Vinokur, A., Van Ryn, M. and Gramlich, L. (1991) 'Long-term follow up benefit cost analysis of the JOBS programme: A preventative intervention for the unemployed', *Journal of Applied Psychology*, vol. 76, pp. 213–19.

Vizard, E., Monck, E. and Misch, P. (1995) 'Child and adolescent sex abuse perpetrators: a review of the research literature', *Journal of Child Psychology and Psychiatry*, vol. 36, pp. 731–56.

von Bertalanffy, L. (1950) 'The theory of open systems in physics and biology', *Science*, vol. 13, pp. 23–9.

von Bertalanffy, L. (1968) *General Systems Theory* (New York: Braziller).

Waddington, J.L., Youssef, H.A. and Kinsella, A. (1998) 'Mortality in schizophrenia. Anti-psychotic polypharmacy and absence of adjunctive anticholinergics over the course of a 10 year prospective study', *British Journal of Psychiatry*, vol. 173, no. 10, pp. 325–29.

Wade, T.J. and Cairney, J. (1997) 'Age and depression in nationally representative sample of Canadians', *Canadian Journal of Public Health*, vol. 88, pp. 297–302.

Wagner, M., Blackorby, J., Cameto, R., Hebbeler, K. and Newman, L. (1993) *The Transition Experiences of Youth with Disabilities* (Palo Alto,CA: SRI).

Walker, M. (1990) *Women in Therapy and Counselling* (Milton Keynes: Open University Press).

Wallace, E.R. (1994) 'Psychiatry and its nosology: an historico-philosophical overview', in J.Z. Sadler, O.P. Wiggins and M.A. Schwartz (eds) *Philosophical Perspectives on Psychiatric Diagnostic Classification* (Baltimore/London: Johns Hopkins University Press).

Wallace, R. and Wallace, D. (1997) 'Socio-economic determinants of health: community marginalisation and the diffusion of disease and disorder in the United States', *British Medical Journal*, vol. 314, p. 1341 (3 May).

Wang, X., Gao, L., Shinfuku, N., Huabiao, Z., Chengshi, Z. and Yucun, S. (2000) 'Longitudinal study of Earthquake related PTSD in a randomly selected community sample in North China', *The American Journal of Psychiatry*, vol. 157, no. 8, pp. 1260–6.

Warner, R. (1985) *Recovery from Schizophrenia: Psychiatry and Political Economy* (London: Routledge).

Weber, J.J., Solomon, M. and Bachrach, H.M. (1985) 'Characteristics of psychoanalytic clinic patients', *International Review of Psychoanalysis*, vol. 12, pp. 13–26.

Weich, S. and Lewis, G. (1998) 'Material standard of living, social class and the prevalence of the common mental disorders in Great Britain', *Journal of Epidemiology and Community Health*, vol. 52, pp. 8–14.

Weich, S., Lewis, G. and Jenkins, S.P. (2001) 'Income inequality and the prevalence of common mental disorders in Britain', *British Journal of Psychiatry*, vol. 179, pp. 222–7.

Weighill, V.E., Hodge, J. and Peck, D.F. (1983) 'Keeping appointments with clinical psychologists', *British Journal of Clinical Psychology*, vol. 22, pp. 143–4.

Westermeyer, J. and Kroll, J. (1978) 'Violence and mental illness in a peasant society: characteristics of violent behaviours and 'folk' use of restraints', *British Journal of Psychiatry*, vol. 133, pp. 529–41.

WHO (1998) *Health for All in the 21st Century* (Copenhagen: World Health Organisation).

Widom, C.P. (1998) 'Childhood victimisation: early adversity and subsequent psychopathology', in B.P. Dohrenwend (ed.) *Adversity, Stress and Psychopathology* (Oxford: Oxford University Press).

Wilden, A. (1972) *System and Structure: Essays in Communication and Exchange* (London: Tavistock).

Wilkinson, R. (2000) *Mind the Gap: Hierarchies, Health and Human Evolution* (London: Weidenfeld & Nicolson).

Wilkinson, R.G. (1996) *Unhealthy Societies: The Afflictions of Inequalities* (London: Routledge).

Wilkinson, R.G., Kawachi, I. and Kennedy, B.P. (1998) 'Mortality, the social environment, crime and violence', *Sociology of Health and Illness*, vol. 20, no. 5, pp. 578–97.

Williams, D. and Harris-Reid, M. (1999) 'Race and Mental Health: emerging patterns and promising approaches' in A. Horwitz and T.L. Scheid (eds) *A Handbook for the Study of Mental Health* (Cambridge: Cambridge University Press).

Williams, J. (1997) *Cry of Pain* (Harmondsworth: Penguin)

Williams, P., Tarnopolosky, A., Hand, D. and Shepherd, M. (1986) 'Minor psychiatric morbidity and general practice consultations: the West London Survey', *Psychological Medicine Monograph*, Supplement 9.

Williams, R. (1983) 'Concepts of health and illness: an analysis of lay logic', *Sociology*, vol. 17, no. 2, pp. 112–26.

Williams, S.J. (1995) 'Theorising class, health and lifestyles: can Bourdieu help us?', *Sociology of Health and Illness*, vol. 17, no. 5, pp. 577–604.

Wing, J. (1978) *Reasoning about Madness* (Oxford: Oxford University Press).

Winnicott, D.W. (1958) *Collected Works* (London: Hogarth Press).

Wittchen, H.U. (2000) 'Epidemiological research in mental disorders: lessons for the next decade of research', the NAPE Lecture 1999, *Acta Psychiatrica Scandinavia*, vol. 101, no. 1, pp. 2–10.

Wolman, B.B. (1968) *Historical Roots of Contemporary Psychology* (New York: Harper Row).

Woolcock, M. (1998) 'Social capital and economic development: toward a theoretical synthesis and policy framework', *Theory and Society*, vol. 27, pp. 151–208.

Wright, B.R.E., Caspi, A., Moffitt, T.E. and Silva, P.A. (1999) 'Low self-control, social bonds, and crime: social causation, social selection or both?', *Criminology*, vol. 37, no. 3, pp. 479–514.

Wright, E.R., Gronfein, W.P. and Owens, T.J. (2000) 'Deinstitutionalization, Social Rejection, and the Self-Esteem of Former Mental Patients (2000)', *Journal of Health and Social Behavior*, vol. 41, pp. 68–90.

Wurtele, S.K. (1999) 'Victims of child maltreatment', in A.S. Bellack and M. Hersen (eds) *Comprehensive Clinical Psychology vol. 9 Applications in Diverse Populations* (London: Pergamon).

Wyatt, G. (1985) 'The sexual abuse of Afro-American and White-American women in Childhood', *Child Abuse and Neglect*, vol. 9, pp. 507–19.

Yamamoto, J., James, Q.C. and Palley, N. (1968) 'Cultural problems in psychiatric therapy', *Archives of General Psychiatry,* vol. 19, pp. 45–49.

Ziegler-Dendy, C.A. (1989) 'The invisible children project: methods and findings', in A. Algarin *et al.* (eds) *Second Annual Conference Proceedings of the Research and Training.*